AF514596

Preventing Age Related Fertility Loss

Dominic Stoop
Editor

Preventing Age Related Fertility Loss

Springer

Editor
Dominic Stoop
Centre for Reproductive Medicine
UZ Brussel
Brussels
Belgium

ISBN 978-3-319-14856-4 ISBN 978-3-319-14857-1 (eBook)
DOI 10.1007/978-3-319-14857-1

Library of Congress Control Number: 2017955781

© Springer International Publishing Switzerland 2018
This work is subject to copyright. All rights are reserved by the Publisher, whether the whole or part of the material is concerned, specifically the rights of translation, reprinting, reuse of illustrations, recitation, broadcasting, reproduction on microfilms or in any other physical way, and transmission or information storage and retrieval, electronic adaptation, computer software, or by similar or dissimilar methodology now known or hereafter developed.
The use of general descriptive names, registered names, trademarks, service marks, etc. in this publication does not imply, even in the absence of a specific statement, that such names are exempt from the relevant protective laws and regulations and therefore free for general use.
The publisher, the authors and the editors are safe to assume that the advice and information in this book are believed to be true and accurate at the date of publication. Neither the publisher nor the authors or the editors give a warranty, express or implied, with respect to the material contained herein or for any errors or omissions that may have been made. The publisher remains neutral with regard to jurisdictional claims in published maps and institutional affiliations.

Printed on acid-free paper

This Springer imprint is published by Springer Nature
The registered company is Springer International Publishing AG
The registered company address is: Gewerbestrasse 11, 6330 Cham, Switzerland

Preface

The age-related fertility loss biologically limits the time for women to successfully conceive and safely carry a pregnancy to term. This limited and individually variable reproductive timespan is especially confronting in view of the continued increase in overall live expectancy and the profoundly altered societal context.

As most fertility specialist around the world, I'm faced with the emotional burden caused by age-related subfertility. In my clinical practice as a fertility specialist at the Centre for Reproductive Medicine in Brussels, I also realized that many, especially single women, are faced with their ticking biological clock and desperate to safeguard (part of) their reproductive potential until they find the right partner.

To my knowledge, this is the first academic book to focus on the different aspects related to this timely topic. I would like to express my deepest gratitude to all the authors for their kind cooperation which made this scientific book possible.

Brussels, Belgium
16 June 2017

Dominic Stoop

Contents

Chapter 1
Female Age and Reproductive Chances

A.C. de Kat and F.J.M. Broekmans

Introduction

We currently live in an era of family planning and female work-force emancipation, while experiencing an ever-increasing lifespan. With this has come the freedom and ability to delay the age of childbearing and facilitate conception. However, for some women this delay may result in having to undergo assisted reproductive treatment (ART) to achieve pregnancy or even in the inability to conceive at all. While calendar, or 'chronological age' is very much related to biological or 'reproductive age', they can also represent separate entities. This means that while some women will be able to achieve a spontaneous pregnancy at age 35 without any problems, others may then have already missed their window of optimal opportunity. This chapter will cover the basic aspects of the reproductive physiology of the aging woman, as well as the demographics and consequences of postponed reproduction.

Physiology of Reproductive Aging

Oocyte Quantity

During the intra-uterine development of a female she is endowed with a supply of egg cells, or oocytes, which is not able to multiply and will thus decrease throughout her reproductive lifespan. The oocytes are surrounded by a layer of granulosa and theca cells, together constituting a follicle. In its earliest stage of development, while in the resting and non-developing pool, the follicle is considered to be

A.C. de Kat (✉) • F.J.M. Broekmans
Reproductive Medicine and Gynaecology, University Medical Center Utrecht,
Heidelberglaan 100, 3508 GA Utrecht, The Netherlands
e-mail: a.c.dekat@umcutrecht.nl

© Springer International Publishing Switzerland 2018

D. Stoop (ed.), *Preventing Age Related Fertility Loss*,
DOI 10.1007/978-3-319-14857-1_1

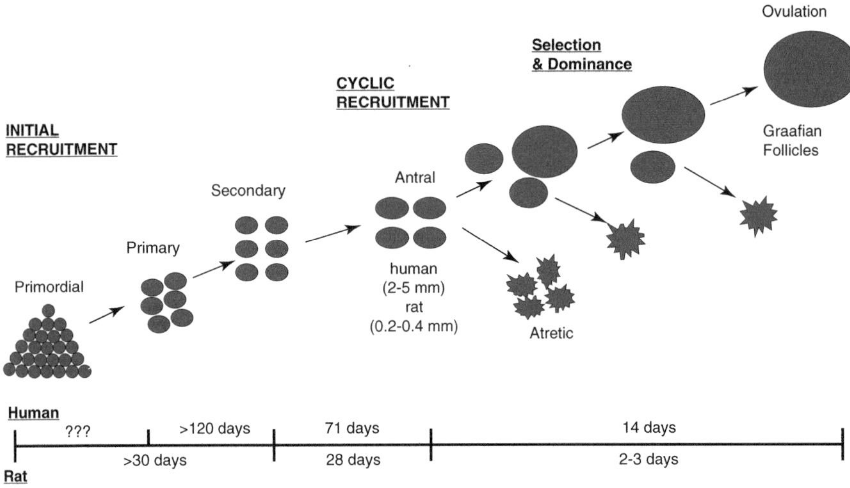

Fig. 1.1 Schematic overview of follicular recruitment and apoptosis

primordial. Starting at birth, follicle numbers in the resting pool decline through apoptosis of the resting follicles. After puberty, primordial follicles are either recruited to undergo development during the menstrual cycle, or go into apoptosis at any stage from resting through development (Fig. 1.1). The vast majority of all ovarian follicles will ultimately be lost through apoptosis [1, 2]. Through these pathways, the follicle pool declines with time, and thus with age.

At around 20 weeks of gestation, the pool of oocytes is fully developed, reaching a number of about seven million [2–4]. At birth, the number of follicles will have already decreased to approximately 1–2 million [4, 5]. With time, the oocyte pool declines further. At menarche, the number of remaining oocytes is thought to be 300,000–400,000 [6], with an estimated 1000 oocytes remaining at the time of menopause [7], marking the end of the female reproductive lifespan. The onset of menopause coincides with the final menstrual period and occurs at an average age of 51 years, with ages between 40 and 60 years considered as the normal variation [4, 8–10].

Oocyte Quality

In addition to a decrease in absolute follicle numbers with time, the aging ovary is also affected by a deterioration of oocyte quality. In the development from a primordial follicle to fertilization, it is necessary for the oocyte to undergo two stages of meiosis in order to reach a haploid state. With advancing female age, the ability of the oocyte to undergo successful and high quality meiosis decreases, as reviewed by Handyside et al. [11]. Experimental mice studies demonstrated increased aneuploidy rates resulting from impaired meiotic divisions of oocytes in long-living females, also known as meiotic non-disjunction, with various causative mechanisms related to errors in the cohesion and division of chromatids [12–15]. In humans, embryonic and fetal aneuploidies due to failures in both the meiosis I and II stages more often stem from aneuploidies in oocytes than spermatozoa [11, 16–18]. In assisted reproduction embryos, the number of aneuploidies exponentially increased with increasing maternal age [19, 20]. The significantly lower aneuploidy rate in older women with donor oocyte pregnancies confirms the aging oocyte to be the most important contributor to aneuploidic pregnancies [21].

Another consequence of female aging for the ovary is the effect on mitochondrial DNA, which is maternally inherited. Mitochondrial DNA functions as a reactive oxygen species (ROS) scavenger and is involved in cell metabolism by generating ATP for several functions [22]. As a woman ages, mitochondrial DNA sustains more damage and an increase in the number of mutations. After meiosis, the oocytes of aging women therefore increasingly contain damaged mitochondrial DNA, with a concomitant decline of total mitochondrial DNA content [22–24].

Besides the intrinsic aspects of aging described above, oocyte quality is also suggested to be influenced by extrinsic factors related to aging such as lifestyle (e.g. smoking [25]), disease and environmental factors and oxidative stress exposure [11, 26]. These factors may cause damage to the oocyte directly, but are also known to influence the epigenetic cell milieu. In animal studies, aging was associated with changes in DNA methylation and histone modification in oocytes, which resulted in an increased aneuploidy rate [27]. Epigenetic modifications are thought to lead to disturbances in the RNA expression necessary for follicular development, changes in the expression of DNA governing the meiosis process, and post-ovulatory DNA modifications [27], which in turn can cause aneuploidy.

The Reproductive Consequences of Biological Aging

Oocyte Quantity Decline

During the development of follicles recruited from the primordial follicle pool, a constant interplay consists between hormones produced by the follicular granulosa cells and those secreted from the hypothalamus and pituitary. This enables the regular cyclic pattern of ovulation and menstruation. When the primordial follicle pool, and thus the number of developing follicles selected from this pool, decrease to a certain threshold, the endocrine balance is altered [28]. Briefly, the relative lack of released gonadal hormones, such as estradiol and inhibin B initiates a mitigated negative feedback signal to the hypothalamus and pituitary, leading to an increase in gonadotrophin-releasing hormone (GnRH). The ensuing higher levels of FSH in combination with the decrease of FSH-sensitive follicles [4] cause dysregulation of follicle development and release. Initially, the increase of FSH-levels gives the development of antral, and selection of dominant, follicles an impulse. This results in an uninhibited dominant follicle selection during the menstrual cycle, which therefore remains regular. With increasing FSH levels, the chance of early, or 'advanced' dominant follicle growth increases [29]. This leads to the shortening of the menstrual cycle, which is the first noticeable sign of decreasing ovarian reserve. Eventually, the relative lack of available antral follicles inhibits the regular selection of a dominant follicle and ovulation, thus leading to an irregular length of the menstrual cycle, marking the beginning of the perimenopausal transition [28, 30]. The irregularity of menstrual cycles becomes more pronounced in the late stage of the perimenopausal transition, which continues until the final menstrual period, heralding the onset of menopause [30]. The time between the onset of irregular cycles and the onset of menopause is thought to be similar for all women, irrespective of their age at menopause (albeit studied in a population of women in which age at menopause ranged between 44 and 55 years) [31].

Oocyte Quality Decline

Although changes in the menstrual cycle pattern are indicative of having reached the later stages of reproductive aging, they will already have been preceded by a decline in fertility. Figure 1.2 summarizes the putative stages of fertility decline with age, from optimal fertility to menopause. At a mean age of 30–31 years, the per-cycle chance of achieving an ongoing pregnancy starts to decrease, due to either impaired fertilization or implantation [32, 33]. Data from a contained, religious community not applying any form of reproductive constriction, in the Québec

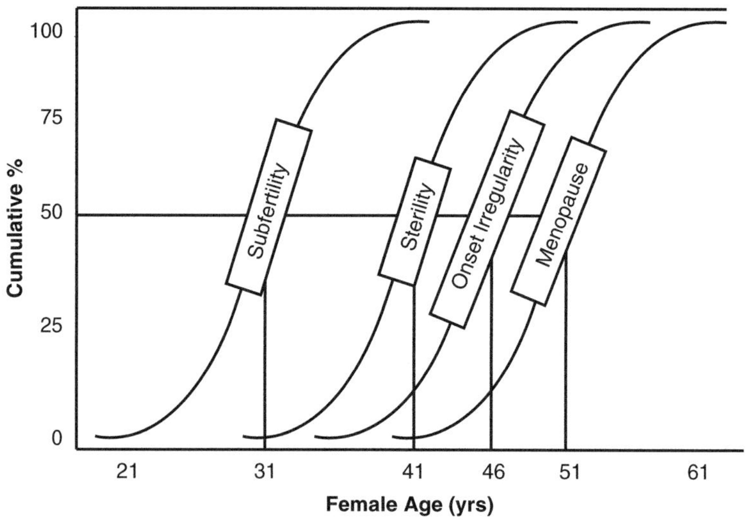

Fig. 1.2 Stages of fertility decline and menstrual cycle changes with increasing female age. Re-used from [6]

region in the early nineteenth century suggest that natural sterility subsequently occurs at an average age of 41 years, with a putative fixed interval of 10 years before the onset of menopause [34]. The occurrence of natural sterility a whole decade before the follicle pool is depleted can be problematic for women delaying their age of conception. It was recently estimated that women who wish to have respectively two or three children through natural conception should start as early as age 27 or 23 in order to have a 90% chance of realizing this objective [35].

The impact of deteriorating oocyte quality on fertility extends further than just fertilization. Miscarriage rates start increasing in women trying to conceive after 30 years of age, and exponentially so after age 35 [36]. The observed miscarriage rates are likely only the tip of the iceberg, as a large number of pregnancies may have miscarried before they could become clinically apparent [6]. Chromosomal abnormalities lie at the heart of at least 50% of all known miscarriages in the general population [37], but even in the event of an ongoing pregnancy, chromosomal abnormalities can still occur. The incidence of trisomy 13, 18 and in particular 21 sharply increases with advancing maternal age [14, 38, 39]. Between the age of 15 and 45, the incidence of a fetus with Down syndrome (trisomy 21) increases from 0.6/1000 to 4.1/1000 [40, 41]. In a large epidemiological study from the United Kingdom, at least 95% of all Down syndrome cases were associated with meiotic non-disjunction [42].

The importance of oocyte quality in addition to quantity is exemplified by a group of women with the same extent of diminished ovarian reserve, wherein younger women had significantly better pregnancy rates [43]. Furthermore, oocyte quantity decline cannot independently predict implantation and pregnancy rates [44]. Male and uterine factors are also an important aspect of fertilization and implantation, but the high pregnancy rates in older women with donated oocytes suggest that the aging oocyte plays a primary role [45].

Measuring Reproductive Aging

Chronological aging does not necessarily follow the same pace as reproductive aging. It can thus be the case that two women of the same chronological age have a very different 'reproductive age' and, as a result, different reproductive chances. A method of quantifying ovarian age was searched for in the field of ART, in order to individualize ovulation induction dosages and estimate the feasibility of fertility treatment.

Oocyte Quantity Markers

The past decade saw the emergence of several markers that represent the size of the remaining primordial follicle pool. Here, we briefly present two such markers frequently used in clinical practice, also known as ovarian reserve tests (ORT): antral follicle count (AFC) and anti-Müllerian hormone (AMH). From the non-growing pool, follicles are continuously selected to develop under the influence of FSH. Although the primordial follicle pool cannot be directly measured, the number of antral follicles, which can be determined by ultrasound, is directly correlated to the number of primordial follicles [46, 47]. Another proxy of the size of the primordial follicle pool is AMH [48], which is produced by the granulosa cells of small developing follicles [49, 50] and can be measured in the peripheral circulation. Both AFC and AMH give an indication of the expected response to ovarian stimulation [51–53], but are also used as markers of the reproductive lifespan. Antral follicle count and AMH concentrations can better predict age at menopause than chronological aging or family history alone, in which respect AMH appears superior to AFC [54]. Predicting the age at which a woman will reach menopause could potentially guide women and clinicians in decisions regarding family planning (when to start having children) and fertility treatment. However, despite initially hopeful results of age at menopause prediction with AMH, it is still not possible to pinpoint an exact age at menopause for an individual woman [54].

Oocyte Quality Markers

In order to provide an estimation of the reproductive chances of women with advanced age, it would be desirable to have a marker of oocyte quality in addition to oocyte quantity. In theory, if the aging processes that influence both oocyte quantity and quality run in parallel, the decline in oocyte quantity could also be a measure of deteriorating oocyte quality. There is some dispute as to whether markers of oocyte quantity are indeed representative oocyte quality. This can be divided into two categories: fecundability, or the per-cycle chance of achieving a pregnancy, and fetal or embryonic aneuploidy. Levels of AMH below 0.7 ng/mL were associated with a 62% reduced chance of achieving pregnancy in an ovulatory cycle [55], but others found no association between ovarian reserve markers and pregnancy rate [56–58] or time to pregnancy [59]. With regard to fetal aneuploidy, there is evidence suggesting that trisomy occurrence is related to reduced AMH levels [60], or decreased ovarian reserve due to congenital ovarian absence or unilateral surgery [61, 62], whereas no association between oocyte quantity and fetal aneuploidy is reported elsewhere [63, 64]. The latter is supported by a study in which embryonic aneuploidy rates were strongly related to maternal age, but not to the number of available embryos per stimulated cycle [19]. In other words, oocyte quantity does not appear to be unequivocally related to oocyte quality. The use of oocyte quantity markers for fertility work-up and counseling may therefore be limited. To date, there are still no known markers that are solely indicative of oocyte quality.

Strategies for Reproduction at Advanced Age

In practice, the majority of women will be able to successfully achieve an ongoing pregnancy. Those who do not and have clear reasons for their sub- or infertility, such as tubal factor, azoospermia, or anovulation may benefit from targeted treatment strategies to their problem. However, when a reduced oocyte quantity or quality lies at the heart of involuntary childlessness, the solution is less simple. To date, there are no known ways to increase oocyte quantity or improve oocyte quality. Treatment for ovarian aging therefore currently has a more preventative nature: women are advised not to postpone a pregnancy for too long and should consider lifestyle habits such as smoking to be a constant threat factor for their (future) fertility. At a late stage of ovarian aging, oocyte donation, using eggs form young or at least previously fertile women, may be the only remaining treatment option for a viable euploidic pregnancy.

Key Message

1. Female aging is associated with a decline in quantity and quality of oocytes.
2. The decline in oocyte quantity ultimately results in the onset of menopause, while the decline in oocyte quality leads to an increased proportion of chromosomal abnormalities.
3. Reproductive aging is associated with a loss in fertility and increase in miscarriage rates.
4. Oocyte quantity can be measured through proxy markers, but there are currently no available markers of oocyte quality.
5. Besides prevention, there are currently no treatment options for the consequences of female reproductive aging.

References

1. Hsueh AJ, Billig H, Tsafriri A. Ovarian follicle atresia: a hormonally controlled apoptotic process. Endocr Rev. 1994;15(6):707–24.
2. te Velde ER, Scheffer GJ, Dorland M, Broekmans FJ, Fauser BC. Developmental and endocrine aspects of normal ovarian aging. Mol Cell Endocrinol. 1998;145(1–2):67–73.
3. Gougeon A, Chainy GB. Morphometric studies of small follicles in ovaries of women at different ages. J Reprod Fertil. 1987;81(2):433–42.
4. Broekmans FJ, Soules MR, Fauser BC. Ovarian aging: mechanisms and clinical consequences. Endocr Rev. 2009;30(5):465–93.
5. Baker TG. A quantitative and cytological study of germ cells in human ovaries. Proc R Soc Lond B Biol Sci. 1963;158:417–33.
6. te Velde ER, Pearson PL. The variability of female reproductive ageing. Hum Reprod Update. 2002;8(2):141–54.

7. Faddy MJ, Gosden RG. A model conforming the decline in follicle numbers to the age of menopause in women. Hum Reprod. 1996;11(7):1484–6.
8. Bengtsson C, Lindquist O, Redvall L. Menstrual status and menopausal age of middle-aged Swedish women. A population study of women in Goteborg 1968–69 and 1974–75. Acta Obstet Gynecol Scand. 1981;60(3):269–75.
9. Treloar AE. Menstrual cyclicity and the pre-menopause. Maturitas. 1981;3(3–4):249–64.
10. Luoto R, Kaprio J, Uutela A. Age at natural menopause and sociodemographic status in Finland. Am J Epidemiol. 1994;139(1):64–76.
11. Handyside AH. Molecular origin of female meiotic aneuploidies. Biochim Biophys Acta. 2012;1822(12):1913–20.
12. Pan H, Ma P, Zhu W, Schultz RM. Age-associated increase in aneuploidy and changes in gene expression in mouse eggs. Dev Biol. 2008;316(2):397–407.
13. Chiang T, Schultz RM, Lampson MA. Age-dependent susceptibility of chromosome cohesion to premature separase activation in mouse oocytes. Biol Reprod. 2011;85(6):1279–83.
14. Kurahashi H, Tsutsumi M, Nishiyama S, Kogo H, Inagaki H, Ohye T. Molecular basis of maternal age-related increase in oocyte aneuploidy. Congenit Anom (Kyoto). 2012;52(1):8–15.
15. MacLennan M, Crichton JH, Playfoot CJ, Adams IR. Oocyte development, meiosis and aneuploidy. Semin Cell Dev Biol. 2015;45:68–76.
16. Hassold T, Hunt PA, Sherman S. Trisomy in humans: incidence, origin and etiology. Curr Opin Genet Dev. 1993;3(3):398–403.
17. Nagaoka SI, Hassold TJ, Hunt PA. Human aneuploidy: mechanisms and new insights into an age-old problem. Nat Rev Genet. 2012;13(7):493–504.
18. Herbert M, Kalleas D, Cooney D, Lamb M, Lister L. Meiosis and maternal aging: insights from aneuploid oocytes and trisomy births. Cold Spring Harb Perspect Biol. 2015;7(4):a017970.
19. Ata B, Kaplan B, Danzer H, Glassner M, Opsahl M, Tan SL, et al. Array CGH analysis shows that aneuploidy is not related to the number of embryos generated. Reprod Biomed Online. 2012;24(6):614–20.
20. Demko ZP, Simon AL, McCoy RC, Petrov DA, Rabinowitz M. Effects of maternal age on euploidy rates in a large cohort of embryos analyzed with 24-chromosome single-nucleotide polymorphism-based preimplantation genetic screening. Fertil Steril. 2016;105(5):1307–13.
21. Kornafel KL, Sauer MV. Increased rates of aneuploidy in older women. Increased rates of aneuploidy do not occur in gestations of older embryo recipients. Hum Reprod. 1994;9(11):1981–2.
22. Hart RJ. Physiological aspects of female fertility: role of the environment, modern lifestyle, and genetics. Physiol Rev. 2016;96(3):873–909.
23. Suganuma N, Kitagawa T, Nawa A, Tomoda Y. Human ovarian aging and mitochondrial DNA deletion. Horm Res. 1993;39(Suppl 1):16–21.
24. Schatten H, Sun QY, Prather R. The impact of mitochondrial function/dysfunction on IVF and new treatment possibilities for infertility. Reprod Biol Endocrinol. 2014;12:111.
25. Tawfik H, Kline J, Jacobson J, Tehranifar P, Protacio A, Flom JD, et al. Life course exposure to smoke and early menopause and menopausal transition. Menopause. 2015;22(10):1076–83.
26. Tarin JJ, Perez-Albala S, Cano A. Oral antioxidants counteract the negative effects of female aging on oocyte quantity and quality in the mouse. Mol Reprod Dev. 2002;61(3):385–97.
27. Ge ZJ, Schatten H, Zhang CL, Sun QY. Oocyte ageing and epigenetics. Reproduction. 2015;149(3):R103–14.
28. Butler L, Santoro N. The reproductive endocrinology of the menopausal transition. Steroids. 2011;76(7):627–35.
29. van Zonneveld P, Scheffer GJ, Broekmans FJ, Blankenstein MA, de Jong FH, Looman CW, et al. Do cycle disturbances explain the age-related decline of female fertility? Cycle characteristics of women aged over 40 years compared with a reference population of young women. Hum Reprod. 2003;18(3):495–501.
30. Soules MR, Sherman S, Parrott E, Rebar R, Santoro N, Utian W, et al. Stages of reproductive aging workshop (STRAW). J Womens Health Gend Based Med. 2001;10(9):843–8.

31. Lisabeth L, Harlow S, Qaqish B. A new statistical approach demonstrated menstrual patterns during the menopausal transition did not vary by age at menopause. J Clin Epidemiol. 2004;57(5):484–96.
32. Schwartz D, Mayaux MJ. Female fecundity as a function of age: results of artificial insemination in 2193 nulliparous women with azoospermic husbands. Federation CECOS. N Engl J Med. 1982;306(7):404–6.
33. van Noord-Zaadstra BM, Looman CW, Alsbach H, Habbema JD, te Velde ER, Karbaat J. Delaying childbearing: effect of age on fecundity and outcome of pregnancy. BMJ. 1991;302(6789):1361–5.
34. Eijkemans MJ, van Poppel F, Habbema DF, Smith KR, Leridon H, te Velde ER. Too old to have children? Lessons from natural fertility populations. Hum Reprod. 2014;29(6):1304–12.
35. Habbema JD, Eijkemans MJ, Leridon H, te Velde ER. Realizing a desired family size: when should couples start? Hum Reprod. 2015;30(9):2215–21.
36. Nybo Andersen AM, Wohlfahrt J, Christens P, Olsen J, Melbye M. Maternal age and fetal loss: population based register linkage study. BMJ. 2000;320(7251):1708–12.
37. Lathi RB, Gray Hazard FK, Heerema-McKenney A, Taylor J, Chueh JT. First trimester miscarriage evaluation. Semin Reprod Med. 2011;29(6):463–9.
38. Hecht CA, Hook EB. Rates of Down syndrome at livebirth by one-year maternal age intervals in studies with apparent close to complete ascertainment in populations of European origin: a proposed revised rate schedule for use in genetic and prenatal screening. Am J Med Genet. 1996;62(4):376–85.
39. Hulten MA, Patel S, Jonasson J, Iwarsson E. On the origin of the maternal age effect in trisomy 21 Down syndrome: the Oocyte Mosaicism Selection model. Reproduction. 2010;139(1):1–9.
40. Cuckle HS, Wald NJ, Thompson SG. Estimating a woman's risk of having a pregnancy associated with Down's syndrome using her age and serum alpha-fetoprotein level. Br J Obstet Gynaecol. 1987;94(5):387–402.
41. Cuckle HS. Primary prevention of Down's syndrome. Int J Med Sci. 2005;2(3):93–9.
42. Mutton D, Alberman E, Hook EB. Cytogenetic and epidemiological findings in Down syndrome, England and Wales 1989 to 1993. National Down Syndrome Cytogenetic Register and the Association of Clinical Cytogeneticists. J Med Genet. 1996;33(5):387–94.
43. Check JH, Cohen R. Evidence that oocyte quality in younger women with diminished oocyte reserve is superior to those of women of advanced reproductive age. Med Hypotheses. 2010;74(2):264–7.
44. Hsu A, Arny M, Knee AB, Bell C, Cook E, Novak AL, et al. Antral follicle count in clinical practice: analyzing clinical relevance. Fertil Steril. 2011;95(2):474–9.
45. Sauer MV, Paulson RJ, Lobo RA. Oocyte donation to women of advanced reproductive age: pregnancy results and obstetrical outcomes in patients 45 years and older. Hum Reprod. 1996;11(11):2540–3.
46. Gougeon A, Ecochard R, Thalabard JC. Age-related changes of the population of human ovarian follicles: increase in the disappearance rate of non-growing and early-growing follicles in aging women. Biol Reprod. 1994;50(3):653–63.
47. Hansen KR, Hodnett GM, Knowlton N, Craig LB. Correlation of ovarian reserve tests with histologically determined primordial follicle number. Fertil Steril. 2011;95(1):170–5.
48. Kevenaar ME, Meerasahib MF, Kramer P, van de Lang-Born BM, de Jong FH, Groome NP, et al. Serum anti-Mullerian hormone levels reflect the size of the primordial follicle pool in mice. Endocrinology. 2006;147(7):3228–34.
49. Jeppesen JV, Anderson RA, Kelsey TW, Christiansen SL, Kristensen SG, Jayaprakasan K, et al. Which follicles make the most anti-Mullerian hormone in humans? Evidence for an abrupt decline in AMH production at the time of follicle selection. Mol Hum Reprod. 2013;19(8):519–27.
50. Broer SL, Broekmans FJ, Laven JS, Fauser BC. Anti-Mullerian hormone: ovarian reserve testing and its potential clinical implications. Hum Reprod Update. 2014;20:688–701.

51. Seifer DB, MacLaughlin DT, Christian BP, Feng B, Shelden RM. Early follicular serum Mullerian-inhibiting substance levels are associated with ovarian response during assisted reproductive technology cycles. Fertil Steril. 2002;77(3):468–71.
52. Broekmans FJ, Kwee J, Hendriks DJ, Mol BW, Lambalk CB. A systematic review of tests predicting ovarian reserve and IVF outcome. Hum Reprod Update. 2006;12(6):685–718.
53. Broer SL, van Disseldorp J, Broeze KA, Dolleman M, Opmeer BC, Bossuyt P, et al. Added value of ovarian reserve testing on patient characteristics in the prediction of ovarian response and ongoing pregnancy: an individual patient data approach. Hum Reprod Update. 2013;19(1):26–36.
54. Depmann M, Broer SL, van der Schouw YT, Tehrani FR, Eijkemans MJ, Mol BW, et al. Can we predict age at natural menopause using ovarian reserve tests or mother's age at menopause? A systematic literature review. Menopause. 2016;23:224–32.
55. Steiner AZ, Herring AH, Kesner JS, Meadows JW, Stanczyk FZ, Hoberman S, et al. Antimullerian hormone as a predictor of natural fecundability in women aged 30–42 years. Obstet Gynecol. 2011;117(4):798–804.
56. van Montfrans JM, van Hooff MH, Huirne JA, Tanahatoe SJ, Sadrezadeh S, Martens F, et al. Basal FSH concentrations as a marker of ovarian ageing are not related to pregnancy outcome in a general population of women over 30 years. Hum Reprod. 2004;19(2):430–4.
57. Ripley M, Lanes A, Leveille MC, Shmorgun D. Does ovarian reserve predict egg quality in unstimulated therapeutic donor insemination cycles? Fertil Steril. 2015;103(5):1170–5. e2
58. Zarek SM, Mitchell EM, Sjaarda LA, Mumford SL, Silver RM, Stanford JB, et al. Is anti-Mullerian hormone associated with fecundability? Findings from the EAGeR Trial. J Clin Endocrinol Metab. 2015;100(11):4215–21.
59. Streuli I, de Mouzon J, Paccolat C, Chapron C, Petignat P, Irion OP, et al. AMH concentration is not related to effective time to pregnancy in women who conceive naturally. Reprod Biomed Online. 2014;28(2):216–24.
60. van der Stroom EM, Konig TE, van Dulmen-den Broeder E, Elzinga WS, van Montfrans JM, Haadsma ML, et al. Early menopause in mothers of children with Down syndrome? Fertil Steril. 2011;96(4):985–90.
61. Freeman SB, Yang Q, Allran K, Taft LF, Sherman SL. Women with a reduced ovarian complement may have an increased risk for a child with Down syndrome. Am J Hum Genet. 2000;66(5):1680–3.
62. Haadsma ML, Mooij TM, Groen H, Burger CW, Lambalk CB, Broekmans FJ, et al. A reduced size of the ovarian follicle pool is associated with an increased risk of a trisomic pregnancy in IVF-treated women. Hum Reprod. 2010;25(2):552–8.
63. Plante BJ, Beamon C, Schmitt CL, Moldenhauer JS, Steiner AZ. Maternal antimullerian hormone levels do not predict fetal aneuploidy. J Assist Reprod Genet. 2010;27(7):409–14.
64. Honorato TC, Henningsen AA, Haadsma ML, Land JA, Pinborg A, Lidegaard O, et al. Follicle pool, ovarian surgery and the risk for a subsequent trisomic pregnancy. Hum Reprod. 2015;30(3):717–22.

Chapter 2
Late Motherhood in Low-Fertility Countries: Reproductive Intentions, Trends and Consequences

Tomáš Sobotka and Éva Beaujouan

Introduction

Delayed parenthood is one of the defining features of the massive transformation of family and reproduction in rich countries [1]. The "contraceptive revolution" that started in the late 1960s, together with relatively easy access to abortion in most countries, have given women and couples an effective control over their pregnancies and contributed to changing family and partnership relations [2]. Young people in Western Europe today are sexually active for more than a decade before becoming parents. Policy concerns about high rates of teenage pregnancies, common in many Western countries a few decades ago [3], have gradually given way to heated debates about late motherhood and ticking biological clock [4, 5]. In the United Kingdom, The Royal College of Obstetricians and Gynaecologists [6] declared later maternal age as an "emerging public health issue" that needs to be thoroughly studied.

Scientific and media debates on delayed motherhood take different angles, reflecting upon the advantages as well as drawbacks of this phenomenon. Some view late parenthood as an opportunity and a positive experience [7]. Older parents may offer children higher living standards and more stable family arrangements, improving their future life chances [8]. Often, delayed parenthood is portrayed as risky, potentially endangering mother's and children's health or leading to involuntary childlessness and demographic decline [9, 10]. Discussions in popular press often blame women (and occasionally men) who wait for "too long,"

T. Sobotka (✉) • É. Beaujouan
Wittgenstein Centre for Demography and Global Human Capital (IIASA, VID/ÖAW, WU), Vienna Institute of Demography (Austrian Academy of Sciences), Welthandelsplatz 2, Level 2, 1020 Vienna, Austria
e-mail: tomas.sobotka@oeaw.ac.at

© Springer International Publishing Switzerland 2018

D. Stoop (ed.), *Preventing Age Related Fertility Loss*, DOI 10.1007/978-3-319-14857-1_2

presenting them as selfish, career-oriented, irresponsible, and breaking the "natural order" [11, 12]. Some of these concerns are justified. It has been repeatedly shown that even well educated women are often poorly informed about female reproductive aging, infertility and the increased risk of pregnancy complications, and they often overestimate the chances of becoming pregnant at higher reproductive ages [13–16].

In this chapter we analyse the shift to later parenthood and review its consequences for children and parents, especially mothers. First we analyse the trends in birth rates at advanced reproductive ages (35+), including trends at very high reproductive ages (50+), which were characterised by a rapid rise in first and second birth rates. We show that a relatively high share of childless women and women with one child aged 35–44 still plan to have a child in the future. Subsequently, we analyse success rates of assisted reproduction at advanced reproductive ages and its role in fuelling the trend towards delayed motherhood. Next we discuss the key drivers of delayed parenthood and its demographic consequences. Finally, we briefly review the consequences of delayed motherhood for pregnancy outcomes, maternal and child health and highlight selected positive consequences of later parenthood for mothers and children, which provide economic and social rationale for late reproduction. Our main focus is on developed countries in Europe, North America, Oceania and East Asia which have experienced a continuing shift to delayed reproduction in the last four decades.

Shifting Childbearing to Advanced Reproductive Ages

The Long-Term Trend Towards Late Motherhood

The trend to later motherhood first started in Western and Northern Europe, the United States, Canada, Australia and Japan in the early 1970s, thus reversing the shift towards earlier first births observed during the post-war baby boom era [17]. Other developed countries and regions followed during the 1980s and 1990s. Recently, the mean age at first birth among women has surpassed 30 in several European countries including Italy and Spain, and in South Korea where it reached 31.1 in 2014, the record-high among rich countries (Fig. 2.1). In the most developed countries the age at starting a family among women has shifted from 22–25 in 1970 to 26–30 in 2014, without showing signs of stabilising or reversing.

In most other world regions women still become mothers early in life, but even many of the less developed countries with high fertility have seen postponement of first marriage and first birth and a decline in adolescent births in the last two decades ([21]: 38). A gradual trend towards delayed motherhood has been reported for many middle-income countries with relatively low fertility, including China, Iran, and the countries of Northern Africa, and Latin America (including Chile, Fig. 2.1) [22, 23].

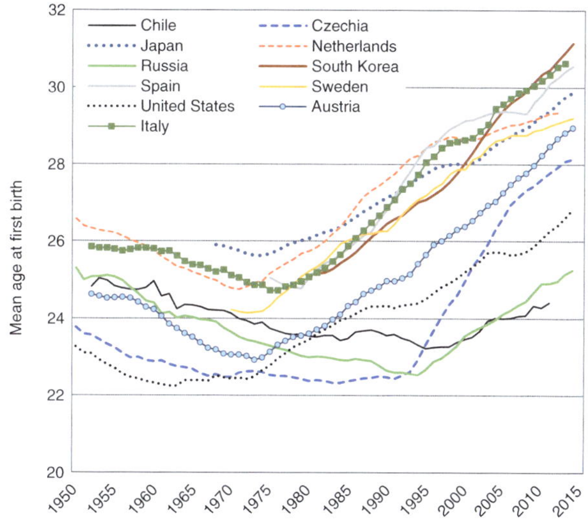

Fig. 2.1 Mean age of women at first birth in selected low-fertility countries, period 1950–2014. Sources: Human Fertility Database [18], Human Fertility Collection [19]. Data for Korea kindly provided by Sam Hyun Yoo [20]

More Frequent Late First and Second Births

Childbearing at higher reproductive ages is not a new phenomenon. Late births had been historically much more common than today, owing to many women having a large family and continuing reproducing until experiencing sterility. In the era of large families until the early twentieth century, childbearing was common even among women past age 40.

With the decline in family size, and a virtual disappearance of large families with more than four children, the historical pattern of having a fourth, fifth or sixth birth at late reproductive ages has been replaced with a new pattern of having a first or a second child later in life. This is especially the case in countries characterized by low fertility rates and a rapid shift to late motherhood, including Italy and Spain. Across the rich low-fertility countries the share of births to women aged 35 and older has risen quickly since 1980 and this increase has been particularly steep for first and second births and at ages 40+ (Table 2.1). For instance, in Japan, the share of first birth rates that took place among women aged 35 and over jumped from 2% in 1980 to 17% in 2014 and the share of second birth rates at these ages jumped from 4 to 26%. At the same time the contribution of women aged 40 and over to total fertility in Japan went up from a low of 0.5 to 3.8% (Table 2.1).

Despite these dramatic shifts, childbearing at ages 40 and higher still remains rather infrequent. In Spain and Sweden, where the shift to late motherhood is well advanced, women gave birth to 0.08 children on average after age 40 in 2014. This amounts to less than 6% of their theoretical reproductive capacity above age 40 estimated at 1.43 children per woman [24]. Late births are even less common in most other rich countries [18].

Table 2.1 Contribution of women aged 35+ and 40+ to total fertility rates (TFR), first birth rates and second birth rates in six developed countries, 1980–2014

	Age 35+			Age 40+		
	Total	First births	Second births	Total	First births	Second births
Japan						
1980	4.3	2.1	3.7	0.5	0.3	0.3
2000	13.3	7.2	14.1	1.5	0.8	1.2
2014	23.0	17.0	25.9	3.8	3.0	3.9
United States						
1980	6.4	1.9	3.9	1.1	0.2	0.4
2000	11.8	6.4	11.5	2.0	1.1	1.7
2014	16.7	9.7	16.6	3.1	1.8	2.7
Netherlands						
1980	6.5	2.1	4.2	1.2	0.3	0.5
2000	16.1	8.6	17.4	2.0	0.9	1.8
2014	19.7	12.0	21.6	2.8	1.7	2.5
Russia						
1980	6.5	1.7	5.4	1.4	0.3	0.7
2000	6.2	2.1	6.7	1.0	0.3	0.8
2014	13.4	4.4	14.9	2.4	0.7	2.2
Spain						
1980	14.0	4.6	7.8	3.7	1.4	1.4
2000	20.2	11.2	25.8	2.8	1.5	2.6
2014	30.3	22.3	38.3	6.1	4.5	6.9
Sweden						
1980	8.4	3.1	6.4	1.3	0.4	0.7
2000	16.3	8.1	15.7	2.6	1.1	2.1
2014	22.1	12.8	22.7	4.1	2.4	3.6

Source: Own computations from the Human Fertility Database [18]

Childbearing at Very High Reproductive Ages

Advances in assisted reproductive technology (ART), especially oocyte cryopreservation, have partly eroded the conventional boundaries of female reproductive lifespan marked by follicular depletion and menopause (see Kat and Broekmans in Chap. 1). In the United States, the number of births to women aged 50+ tripled from 255 in 2000 to 743 in 2014 [25, 26]. In the European Union countries (including the United Kingdom) the number of births to women aged 50+ in 2002–2014 jumped from 287 to 1019 ([27], own computations). Wikipedia [28] provides an extensive list of women who gave birth at age 50 or older, with the three oldest mothers reportedly being all from India and giving birth at age 70 between 2008 and 2016. The oldest mother with fully verified age is Maria del Carmen Bousada from Spain who gave birth to twin boys shortly before her 67th birthday, after receiving ART using donor oocytes in the United States.

Childbearing Intentions and Their Realisation at Higher Reproductive Ages

High Share of Childless Women Aged 35+ Intends to Have a Child

The *Generations and Gender Surveys* (GGS) for six European countries that took place in the 2000s reveal that many women still plan to have a child at an age when their reproductive capacity is declining [29]. This is especially the case in Austria, France, Italy, and Russia where 28–32% of women aged 35–39 intended having a(nother) child (Fig. 2.2). Perhaps more surprising is that more than one in ten women aged 40–44 in Austria, Italy and Russia intended having a(nother) child. These shares were much lower in Czechia and Poland, two post-communist countries where reproduction took place at relatively young ages until the 1990s. However, women at older reproductive ages also express uncertainty about their plans: in each analysed country the share of women responding they "probably" intend to have a child outnumbers the share responding they are "certain" about their intention.

Another consistent finding is a strong family size gradient in reproductive intentions: the plan to have a child later in life is very common among childless women aged 35–39, with a majority of these women intending to become mothers. Also many women with one child still planned to have a second child in the future. In contrast, only a few women having two or more children intended to have another child at later ages (Fig. 2.2b). Very similar gradient is found also for women aged 40–44 and for men at advanced reproductive ages (not shown here; see [30]).

Actual Fertility at Higher Reproductive Ages Matches More Closely the Earlier Reproductive Intentions Among Mothers Than Those Among the Childless

How are intentions to have children later in life related to the actual fertility rates at higher reproductive ages? For three European countries, Austria, Italy, and the Netherlands, we compared survey data on reproductive intentions with the aggregate data on childbearing probabilities by age and parity included in the Human Fertility Database [18] and Human Fertility Collection [19]. We did not follow up

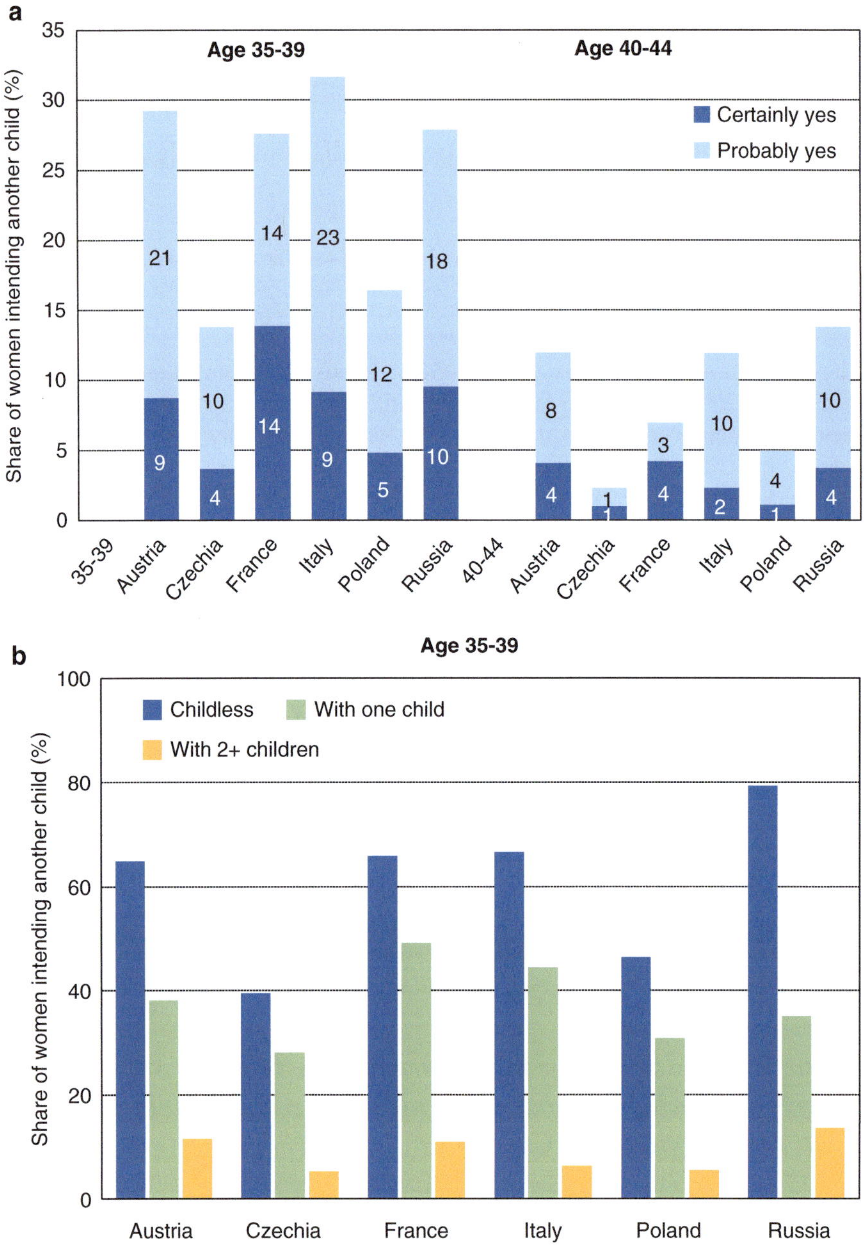

Fig. 2.2 (**a**) Share of women aged 35–39 and 40–44 stating they intend to have a(nother) child in the future; six European countries, surveys organized in 2000s. (**b**) Share of women aged 35–39 stating they intend to have a(nother) child in the future by the number of children they already have; six European countries. The graph combines "probably yes" and "certainly yes" answers. Source: Own computations from the Generations and Gender Survey (GGS) data for Austria 2008–2009, Czechia 2004–2005, France 2005, Italy 2003–2004, Poland 2010–2011, Russia 2004 (see [29] for questions asked and for more details about the data)

Table 2.2 Percentage of Italian women aged 35–39 and 40–44 intending to have a(nother) child (Multiscopo survey in 2009) and the share of women giving birth to a child in the following years (population-level statistics, in percent)

	2009 Multiscopo survey				Population-level fertility data	
	Intention to have a child, %			N	Share having a child (% of all women irrespective of their intention)	Share having a child related to the share intending
	Yes	Probably yes	Total			
Age 35–39						
Childless	24	40	64	463	31	0.48
1 child	14	34	49	411	33	0.67
2+ children	2	10	12	764	9	0.75
Total	12	25	37	1638	22	0.59
Age 40–44						
Childless	7	27	34	362	7	0.20
1 child	3	14	17	436	6	0.33
2+ children	1	1	2	967	1	0.60
Total	3	10	13	1765	4	0.28

Source: Own computations from Multiscopo ISTAT—Family and Social Subjects (2009) survey

the women interviewed at the time of the survey, but we compared their plans with population-wide data on the likelihood of having a child by the end of their reproductive life among all women who were of the same age and had the same number of children in the year intention estimates were calculated.

Table 2.2 illustrates this correspondence for Italy, where 37% of women aged 35–39 intended to have a child in the future (including those saying "probably yes") according to the 2009 Multiscopo survey. This compares with the aggregate data showing that 22% of women of that age gave birth in the years following the survey. A similar correspondence is found for Austria (24% intended to have a child vs. 15% have had a child; see [30], Table 2.2a) and yet closer relationship is found for the Netherlands (20% vs. 16%) (results for Austria and the Netherlands not shown here). These comparisons indicate that women aged 35–39 wishing to have a child in the future still have a relatively good chance of achieving their goal, even when taking into account that those giving birth to a child are not always those who intended to have one.

The gap between reproductive intentions and actual pregnancies becomes much wider at later ages, 40–44, when many women are infertile and the potential mothers often widely overestimate their chances of becoming pregnant (see data for Italy in Table 2.2). In addition, childless women aged 35+ consistently show a larger gap between their reproductive intentions and subsequent childbearing. This gap is partly related to considerable uncertainty about the reproductive plans reported by these women, but it is also due to their unrealistic expectations and adverse life circumstances (which often include not having a partner). Selectivity plays a role as well, with more frequent health problems and higher infertility among the childless.

Assisted Reproduction and Delayed Childbearing

Rising ART Use and Declining ART Success Rates at Higher Reproductive Ages

Many women planning to have a child in their late 30s and early 40s are likely to face infertility and turn to ART treatment. This trend is partly fuelled by widespread misperceptions about the ability of ART to compensate for infertility at later reproductive ages [31], giving women an illusion of fertility control at higher reproductive ages [32, 33]. Despite many rich countries not subsidizing ART for women after a certain age threshold, the number of ART cycles is rising fastest at age 40 and higher. In the United States, 21% of all ART cycles in 2013 (i.e., 34 thousand cycles) were initiated by women aged 41+ (own computations from the Centers for Disease Control and Prevention data [34]).

In Europe, the incomplete data show that the number of registered ART cycles at ages 40+ increased much faster in 2002–2012, by a factor of 3.1, than the number of cycles initiated by younger women, which increased by a factor of 1.8 (computations based on [35, 36]). Especially steep rise was reported for ART using donor oocytes, which quadrupled in the same period. Overall, the share of ART cycles initiated by women aged 40+ jumped from 12 to 19% in 2002–2012, contributing about 7% of all children born to women over age 40.

Success rates of non-donor assisted reproduction, measured especially by the percentage of ART cycles that result in pregnancies and live births or single-infant live births, decline rapidly with age among women past age 32 ([34], Fig. 14). Figure 2.3 illustrates this pattern using the data for the United States. Among women undergoing non-donor ART in 2013, pregnancy rates per cycle reached 46% at ages below 35, 25% at age 40 and only 4% at ages 45+. Because of high rates of miscarriage at higher ages, the fall in the likelihood of live birth following ART cycle is even steeper with age: 40% of non-donor ART cycles initiated at ages <35 resulted in live birth in 2013, compared with 17% of the cycles initiated at age 40 and 2% at ages 45+ (Fig. 2.3). The likelihood of live birth has improved only gradually among women past age 40. A majority of women do not achieve pregnancy leading to live birth after age 40 even after six or more ART cycles [37, 38].

Conventional ART using non-donor oocytes therefore cannot offset age-related fertility decline and for many women it does not provide a realistic chance of having a child after age 40 [31, 39, 40]. Also the cost of ART treatments per live birth delivery rises steeply after age 40, making conventional non-donor ART use problematic, especially after age 45 [41].

In contrast, ART with donor oocytes shows remarkably stable success rate with age of women treated, with the percentage of ART cycles resulting in live births staying over 50% even for women in their 40s according to the US data for 2013 ([34]: Fig. 40) (for more details on treatment options see Drakopoulos and Polyzos in Chap. 3). Therefore, despite higher costs and despite the fact that in case of successful treatment the child will not be genetically related to the mother, the use of donor oocytes increases rapidly. In the United States, donor oocytes accounted for

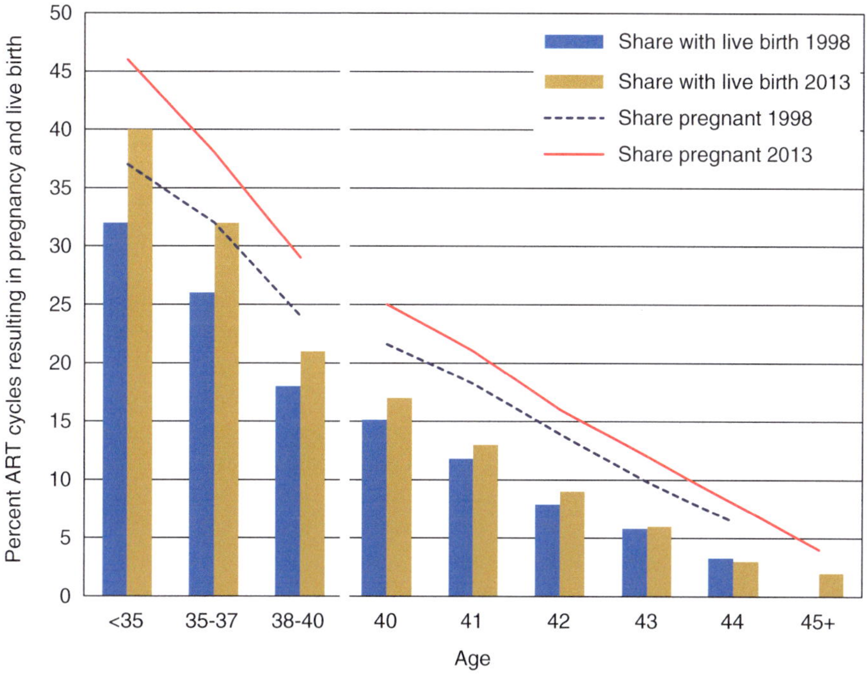

Fig. 2.3 Success rates of ART cycles with non-donor oocytes or embryos by age in the United States: Percentage of cycles resulting in pregnancies and live birth, 1998 and 2013. Source: [34] (Figs. 15 and 17) and 2000 (Figs. 10 and 12). Note: Data for single years of age published only for ages 40–44

37% of ART cycles among women aged 41+ and for around 78% of live births among ART users of that age; for Europe the corresponding estimates were 17% and 41%, respectively (own computations from [34] data and [35] data). In addition, the cryopreservation of oocytes has rapidly evolved and reached the stage when it has become widely available ([42]; see also Chap. 8 and other chapters in this volume). In the US, the number of oocyte or embryo banking cycles rose dramatically from around a thousand in 2006 to over 27 thousand in 2013 [34]. Surprisingly many of these freezing cycles, 30%, are taking place at ages 41+, i.e., at ages when the quality of oocytes deteriorates rapidly, implying lower chances of successful pregnancy and delivery later in life.

Main Factors Contributing to Later Parenthood

A review by Mills et al. [43] identified the following key drivers of the shift towards later parenthood: expanding education, increased employment among women, economic uncertainty and precarious forms of employment, low availability and high costs of housing, delayed and more unstable partnerships, more individualized values including higher acceptance of childlessness, and lower levels of gender equality. These factors often reinforce each other and their importance differs by country and time period [17]. The shift towards later parenthood was supported by widely available efficient contraception, especially the pill [44, 45] and, more recently, by the spread of "emergency contraception" that is used especially among young adult women [46].

Being in education is commonly perceived as incompatible with parenthood [47]. The continuing expansion of higher education in the rich countries during the last four decades has been repeatedly identified as a central driver of delayed parenthood [48, 49]. However, in many countries including the United States, United Kingdom and Norway, highly educated women increasingly shifted childbearing well beyond the time of completing their education, often towards their mid- or late-30s [50–52]. This leads to rising contrasts ("polarization") in first birth timing by social status, especially in Southern Europe and in English-speaking countries [53]. Unemployment and unstable economic conditions have been documented as important factors especially in Southern Europe, where policies supporting family formation are weak and many young adults face precarious labour market situation [54]. At an individual level, not having a suitable partner and, more generally, "not feeling ready" for motherhood are frequently cited as important reasons for delaying motherhood [55, 56].

Demographic Consequences of Delayed Childbearing

The shift to later motherhood has important population-level consequences. It negatively affects period birth rates as some women who would otherwise have had a child in any given year shifted their childbearing plans towards the future. As a result, period total fertility rates are depressed and often decline well below the corresponding indicators of cohort family size [57, 58]. Delayed childbearing implies wider age distance between generations, which in turn means that women and men having children later in life are less likely to survive to see their grandchildren when compared with younger parents or they might not remain in good health when becoming grandparents [59, 60]. The stretched intergenerational interval also implies a slower pace of population decline when fertility rates are below the replacement-level threshold of around 2.07 children per woman in low-mortality countries [61].

Later motherhood can also result in higher childlessness and reduced family size in the population. Leridon and Slama [62] simulated the impact of a postponement of the first pregnancy attempt by 30 and 69 months, initially starting at age 25 on average. The shift by 69 months would reduce the final number of children per woman by more than 10% (from 2.00 to 1.77) and would increase the share of childless couples from 11.7 to 17.7%. Te Velde et al. [63] used similar micro-simulation models, estimating that first birth postponement in six European countries between 1970 and 2007 led to an increase in permanent childlessness in the range of 4% in Czechia to 7% in Spain.

Delayed childbearing is closely associated with higher frequency of multiple births. Their increase with age of the mother is attributable to higher multiple follicle growth with age [64] and to high rates of multiple births following ART. In the highly developed countries the frequency of twin deliveries increased rapidly between 1970 and 2013, typically doubling, but in some cases (Greece, Hong Kong) tripling during that period [65]. In the United States, the number of twin live births per thousand live births went up from 18.9 in 1980 to 33.9 in 2014 ([25], Table 27). The analysis of data for 32 countries by Pison et al. [65] shows that ART use was the main reason for the rising frequency of twin births, contributing on average to three quarters of their observed rise between 1970 and 2005. As single embryo transfers are increasingly preferred by health professionals, the guidelines regulating ART use are being revised. Consequently, the frequency of twin and triplet deliveries peaked in 13 countries including Nordic countries, Australia, Japan, the Netherlands and Japan between 1998 and 2010 and then started declining [65–69].

Consequences of Delayed Motherhood for Pregnancy Outcomes, Maternal and Child Health

Extensive medical literature documents the effects of pregnancy and childbearing at advanced reproductive ages on pregnancy outcomes, foetal development, and maternal and child health (e.g., [60, 70–74]). Many risks are related to "natural pregnancies", but some including multiple deliveries are more typical for ART use. We give only brief highlights of the most important findings; more details are discussed elsewhere in this volume.

Pregnancy complications and foetal loss are more frequent at higher maternal ages. The frequency of miscarriages (spontaneous abortions), ectopic pregnancies as well as stillbirths increases rapidly with age among women in their late 30s and older [60, 75]. Danish register-based study found that at age 42 and older, more than half of pregnancies intended to be carried to term (i.e. excluding induced abortions) resulted in foetal loss, compared with 13.5% of pregnancies across all ages [75]. Male partner's age was also found to be an independent risk factor for miscarriage [76]. Interestingly, women using donor oocytes do not show an increase rise in pregnancy loss with age [77, 78], which again suggests that the age and quality of oocytes are the main factors determining reproductive success (see also Kat and Broekmans in Chap. 1). A combination of rising infertility and more frequent pregnancy losses with age implies that women who have a strong childbearing desire and a preference for larger family should aim to have children relatively early in life. Habbema et al. [79] showed that women planning only one child and willing to take a 50% risk that they do not succeed can start their pregnancy attempt at age 41 (or 42 if they are willing to use ART). Those planning three kids and wanting to have a 90% chance they succeed should start as early as at age 23.

Advanced maternal age is also a risk factor in preterm births [80, 81] and complications during pregnancy and delivery, including high rate of Caesarean delivery, excessive labour bleeding, and higher frequency of diabetes and chronic and pregnancy-induced hypertension among mothers [71, 73, 74]. Older mothers are more likely to suffer from obesity, take medication or experience morbidity (see [82] for obesity). Multiple births, more common at later childbearing ages, constitute an additional risk factor associated with low birth weight of infants, pregnancy complications, maternal risks, and higher long-term morbidity [83, 84]. Among children, advanced maternal age is often linked to higher incidence of congenital anomalies and chromosomal aberrations, as discussed in Chap. 1 by Kat and Broekmans.

Positive Consequences of Parenthood at Later Ages for Parents and Children

The Economic Rationale of Parenthood at Later Ages

Among higher educated women with better-paid jobs and good career prospects there is a strong economic rationale for delaying parenthood well beyond the period of completing education. It is based on a need for couples to accumulate resources before family formation, to have enough resources to rear their children and support their education as they grow up, to qualify for paid maternity and parental leaves, and to minimize the income loss linked to childcare-related career break.

Achieving financial security is often cited by couples as one of the most important factors in their parenthood decisions [16]. In many countries, especially in Southern and Eastern Europe, rental housing is scarce or too costly. Young couples may need to accumulate considerable savings and achieve a stable income before purchasing their own flat or a house—which is often seen as a precondition to having children [85, 86]. Married couples living in US cities with highest rents and housing sales prices were having their first child by 3–4 years later than the couples living in metropolitan areas with cheap housing [87]. In addition, raising children is costly, especially in countries where costs of childcare, healthcare and education shouldered by parents are high. In the US, the cost of raising a child from childbirth up to age 18 was estimated at 245,000 US Dollars for middle-income families, based on the 2013 computations by US Department of Agriculture [88]. This again motivates couples to put off childbearing until both partners achieve stable employment and steady income.

In countries which provide paid maternity and parental leave, including Nordic countries, their level is often linked to pre-leave income and a minimum period of uninterrupted employment before the leave. As this policy is focused on compensating parents their foregone earnings, it motivates prospective parents to get established on the labour market and achieve a stable full-time position before having a child, potentially delaying their parenthood [89]. Finally, among mothers with higher socio-economic position, earning losses due to childcare leave are substantially lower at higher childbearing ages when they are more advanced in their careers, have more secure employment, and experience lower skill depreciation [90–92]. The US data analysed by Herr [93] show that fertility delays are paying off especially for college graduates: for them, each year of delaying motherhood after their labour market entry implies a 2.9% increase in their wage after a 20-year period, accounting for 5.5% of their total wage growth.

Non-economic Positive Consequences of Delayed Parenthood

The positive consequences of delayed parenthood extend beyond resource accumulation, more stable careers and lower income losses. However, the research in this area is relatively limited and the evidence so far is often based on small datasets or data pertaining to one country. Many papers do not address selection effects—the fact that older mothers are also, on average, better educated and healthier, and therefore the possible effects of late motherhood reported below might be more closely associated with their education and health rather than age [94, 95]. Therefore, these findings do not imply causality and have to be interpreted with caution.

Later parenthood is linked with a lower likelihood for children to be born to a mother living without a partner [60] and a lower percentage of unintended pregnancies and births [96, 97]. Children born to older parents experience less frequent parental separation [98] and therefore they also experience living with a single mother or with stepparents less often than the children born earlier in life. The research on three indicators of child's cognitive and behavioural outcomes at the age of three summarised by Hansen et al. [99] showed these outcomes peaking among children born to mothers in their 30s. While much of this developmental advantage was attributable to their mothers' higher education, the positive effect of later motherhood persisted even when mothers' education, return to employment and childcare use were controlled for. Myrskylä and Margolis [100] found that parents at older ages (35+) show more positive happiness trajectory after the childbirth than the younger parents.

Barclay and Myrskylä [101], working with Swedish data, demonstrated additional benefit of late motherhood for children. Children born to older mothers are also born in a later time period, reaping the benefits of improving social conditions over time. They are taller, more likely to attend university and perform better at standardised tests than their siblings born when their mothers were younger. Among mothers, late age at childbearing is associated with better health and longevity [102, 103]. These findings again suggest that some of the benefits of later motherhood might be explained by selectivity of mothers who are fertile (and presumably healthyier) at later ages.

Discussion: The Contrasting Biological and Social Rationales for and Against Late Parenthood

As longevity continues rising, life courses of men and women stretch and they experience many important transitions later in life [104]. They complete their education, move from parental home, enter the labour market, or retire at ever higher ages. The fast increase in the number of women who are childless past age 35 and plan to have a child in the future appears perfectly in line with this trend. With some simplification, children born to older parents are also born to more stable, happier and wealthier families. Many social and economic rationales speak for having children late in life. However, these rationales clash with "inconvenient biology" [105] as there is also a clear biological and health rationale for having children much earlier in life [9, 106]. The steep rise in the number of ART cycles at later reproductive ages illustrates the scale of infertility and unfulfilled pregnancy desires among women who arguably postponed parenthood for too long.

The rise of ART with donor oocytes and the advances in "social egg freezing" have gradually eroded the biological limits to fertility marked by follicular depletion and menopause. The number of post-menopausal women getting pregnant is increasing fast, although from very low numbers. At the same time, a vast majority of women still plan to get pregnant without the help of medically assisted reproduction. They are often caught between the conflicting motivations for and against having children and struggling with the ever more pertinent question of "How long can you wait to have a baby?" [4, 5, 107]. As Habbema et al. [79] demonstrate, the answer depends on family size preferences and the strength of these preferences.

Key Messages

1. A sharp increase in the number of women having their first or second birth after age 35 has taken place across the highly developed countries. Also the frequency of motherhood among post-menopausal women past age 50 is rising fast, but from extremely low levels.
2. Childbearing intentions past age 35 are especially common among the childless women, many of whom will face infertility when trying to realise these plans.
3. Assisted reproduction use has been rising faster among women past age 40 than among the younger age groups. However, success rates of ART using fresh non-donor oocytes remain low at ages 41+, with ART using donor oocytes or women's own cryopreserved oocytes being much more effective and rapidly expanding alternatives.
4. The massive expansion of university education is the main factor behind the shift to later motherhood, followed by unstable labour market and deteriorating economic position of young adults as well as rapid changes in partnership behaviour and the availability of highly efficient contraception.
5. Prospective parents face conflicting rationales for having children earlier or later in life. Biological and health rationales for early childbearing clash with economic and well-being rationales for later reproduction, which include higher family stability and higher happiness among older parents.

Acknowledgments The research by T. Sobotka was funded by the European Research Council under the European Union's Seventh Framework Programme (FP7/2007-2013)/ERC Grant agreement no 284238 (EURREP project). E. Beaujouan's contribution was funded by the Austrian Science Fund (FWF), project FWF P28071-G22 ("Running Against the Clock? Realising Family Plans Over the Life-course"). The earlier more extensive draft of this chapter is available as a working paper [30].

References

1. Lesthaeghe R. The unfolding story of the Second Demographic Transition. Popul Dev Rev. 2010;36(2):211–51.
2. van de Kaa DJ. On the societal impact of modern contraception. In: Beets G, Schippers J, te Velde E, editors. The future of motherhood in western societies. Dordrecht: Springer; 2011. p. 49–60.
3. Jones EF, Forrest JD, Goldman N, Henshaw SK, Lincoln R, Rosoff JI, Westoff CF, Wulf D. Teenage pregnancy in developed countries: determinants and policy implications. Fam Plan Perspect. 1985;17(2):53–63.
4. Heffner LJ. Advanced maternal age—how old is too old? N Engl J Med. 2004;351(19):1927–9.
5. TwengeJ.Howlongcanyouwaittohaveababy?TheAtlanticJuly/August2013Issue.http://www.theatlantic.com/magazine/archive/2013/07/how-long-can-you-wait-to-have-a-baby/309374/
6. Royal College of Obstetricians and Gynaecologists. RCOG statement on later maternal age. 2009. http://www.rcog.org.uk/what-we-do/campaigning-and-opinions/statement/rcog-statement-latermaternal-age
7. La Liberte A. Why have a child after 40? Blog Post. 2012. http://achildafter40.com/about-a-child-after-40/. Accessed Oct 2016.
8. McLanahan S. Diverging destinies: How children are faring under the second demographic transition? Demography. 2004;41(4):607–27.
9. Bewley S, Davies M, Braude P. Which career first? BMJ. 2005;331:588–9.
10. Selvaratnam T. The big lie: motherhood, feminism, and the reality of the biological clock. Amherst, NY: Prometheus Books; 2014.
11. Budds K, Locke A, Burr V. Risky business: constructing the 'choice' to 'delay' motherhood in the British press. Fem Med Stud. 2013;13(1):132–47.
12. Shaw RL, Giles DC. Motherhood on ice? A media framing analysis of older mothers in the UK news. Psychol Health. 2009;24(2):221–36.
13. Bretherick KL, Fairbrother N, Avila L, Harbord SH, Robinson WP. Fertility and aging: do reproductive-aged Canadian women know what they need to know? Fertil Steril. 2010;93(7):2162–8.
14. Daniluk JC, Koert E, Cheung A. Childless women's knowledge of fertility and assisted human reproduction: identifying the gaps. Fertil Steril. 2012;97(2):420–6.
15. Lampic C, Svanberg AS, Karlström P, Tydén T. Fertility awareness, intentions concerning childbearing, and attitudes towards parenthood among female and male academics. Hum Reprod. 2006;21(2):558–64.
16. Tough S, Benzies K, Fraser-Lee N, Newburn-Cook C. Factors influencing childbearing decisions and knowledge of perinatal risks among Canadian men and women. Matern Child Health J. 2007;11(2):189–98.
17. Sobotka T. Postponement of childbearing and low fertility in Europe. Ph.D. Thesis, University of Groningen. Amsterdam: Dutch University Press; 2004.
18. Human Fertility Database. Period and cohort fertility rates by age and birth order; data on mean age at first birth accessed at www.humanfertility.org (data downloaded 5 October 2016). Max Planck Institute for Demographic Research (Germany) and Vienna Institute of Demography (Austria). 2016.

19. Human Fertility Collection. Period age-specific fertility rates accessed at www.fertilitydata.org (data downloaded 5 October 2016). Max Planck Institute for Demographic Research (Germany) and Vienna Institute of Demography (Austria). 2016.
20. Yoo SH, Sobotka T. The role of tempo effect in the ultra-low fertility in South Korea. Paper presented at the 2016 annual meeting of the Population Association of America, Washington, D.C., 1 April 2016, 2016.
21. United Nations. World fertility report 2013: fertility at the extremes. New York: United Nations, Department of Economic and Social Affairs, Population Division; 2013.
22. Rosero-Bixby L, Castro-Martín T, Martín-García T. Is Latin America starting to retreat from early and universal childbearing? Demogr Res. 2009;20(9):169–94.
23. Sobotka T. Post-transitional fertility: the role of childbearing postponement in fuelling the shift to low and unstable fertility levels. J Biosoc Sci. 2017. Forthcoming.
24. Sheps MC. An analysis of reproductive patterns in an American isolate. Popul Stud. 1965;19(1):65–80.
25. Hamilton BE, Martin JA, Osterman MJK et al.. Births: final data for 2014. National vital statistics reports, vol. 64, No. 12. Hyattsville, MD: National Center for Health Statistics; 2015.
26. Martin JA, Hamilton BE, Ventura SJ, Menacker F, Park MM. Births: final data for 2000 national vital statistics reports, vol. 50, No. 5. Hyattsville, MD: National Center for Health Statistics; 2002.
27. Eurostat. Data on births by age of mother and birth order in 2000–2014. Eurostat online database, theme "Population and Social Conditions". 2016. http://ec.europa.eu/eurostat/data/database. Accessed Oct 2016.
28. Wikipedia. Pregnancy over age 50. 2016. https://en.wikipedia.org/wiki/Pregnancy_over_age_50. Accessed 10 Oct 2016.
29. Beaujouan É. Counting how many children people want: The influence of question filters and pre-codes. Demográfia. 2014;56(5):35–61. English edition 2013
30. Beaujouan É, Sobotka T. Late motherhood in low-fertility countries: reproductive intentions, trends and consequences. In: Vienna Institute of Demography Working Papers and Human Fertility Database Research Report VID WP 02/2017 and HFD RR-2017-002; 2017.
31. Wyndham N, Figueira PGM, Patrizio P. A persistent misperception: assisted reproductive technology can reverse the "aged biological clock". Fertil Steril. 2012;97(5):1044–7.
32. Mac Dougall K, Beyene Y, Nachtigall RD. Age shock: misperceptions of the impact of age on fertility before and after IVF in women who conceived after age 40. Hum Reprod. 2012;28(2):350–6.
33. Szewczuk E. Age-related infertility: a tale of two technologies. Sociol Health Illn. 2012;34(3):429–43.
34. CDC. Assisted reproductive technology national summary report 2013. Atlanta (GA): Centers for Disease Control and Prevention, American Society for Reproductive Medicine, Society for Assisted Reproductive Technology, US Dept of Health and Human Services; 2015.
35. Calhaz-Jorge C, De Geyter C, Kupka MS, De Mouzon J, Erb K, Mocanu E, Motrenko T, Scaravelli G, Wyns C, Goossens V, Gliozheni O. Assisted reproductive technology in Europe, 2012: results generated from European registers by ESHRE. Hum Reprod. 2016;31(8):1638–52.
36. Nyboe Andersen A, Gianaroli L, Felberbaum R, de Mouzon J, Nygren KG. Assisted reproductive technology in Europe, 2002. Results generated from European registers by ESHRE. Hum Reprod. 2006;21(7):1680–97.
37. Gnoth C, Maxrath B, Skonieczny T, Friol K, Godehardt E, Tigges J. Final ART success rates: a 10 years survey. Hum Reprod. 2011;26(8):2239–46.
38. Malizia BA, Hacker MR, Penzias AS. Cumulative live-birth rates after in vitro fertilization. N Engl J Med. 2009;360(3):236–43.
39. Leridon H. Can assisted reproduction technology compensate for the natural decline in fertility with age? A model assessment. Hum Reprod. 2004;19(7):1549–54.

40. Ng EHY, Ho PC. Ageing and ART: a waste of time and money? Best Pract Res Clin Obstet Gynaecol. 2007;21(1):5–20.
41. Sullivan E, Wang Y, Chapman M, Chambers G. Success rates and cost of a live birth following fresh assisted reproduction treatment in women aged 45 years and older, Australia 2002–2004. Hum Reprod. 2008;23(7):1639–43.
42. Stoop D, Cobo A, Silber S. Fertility preservation for age-related fertility decline. Lancet. 2014;384(9950):1311–9.
43. Mills M, Rindfuss RR, McDonald P, te Velde E. Why do people postpone parenthood? Reasons and social policy incentives. Hum Reprod Update. 2011;17(6):848–60.
44. Goldin C, Katz LF. The power of the pill: Oral contraceptives and women's career and marriage decisions. J Polit Econ. 2002;110(4):730–70.
45. Bailey MJ. Reexamining the impact of family planning programs on US fertility: Evidence from the War on Poverty and the early years of Title X. Am Econ J Appl Econ. 2012;4(2):62–97.
46. Daniels K, Jones J, Abma J. Use of emergency contraception among women aged 15–44: United States, 2006–2010. NCHS data brief no 112. 2013. Hyattsville, MD: National Center for Health Statistics.
47. Blossfeld H-P, Huinink J. Human capital investments or norms of role transition? How women's schooling and career affect the process of family formation. Am J Sociol. 1991;97(1):143–68.
48. Kalwij A, Gustafsson S, editors. Education and postponement of maternity: economic analyses for industrialized countries. Dordrecht: Kluwer/Springer; 2006.
49. Ní Bhrolcháin M, Beaujouan É. Fertility postponement is largely due to rising educational enrolment. Popul Stud. 2012;66(3):311–27.
50. Berrington A, Stone J, Beaujouan É. Educational differences in timing and quantum of childbearing in Britain: a study of cohorts born 1940–1969. Demogr Res. 2015;33(Article 26):733–64.
51. Lappegård T, Rønsen M. The multifaceted impact of education on entry into motherhood. Eur J Popul. 2005;21(1):31–49.
52. Rindfuss RR, Morgan SP, Offut K. Education and the changing age pattern of American fertility. Demography. 1996;33(3):277–90.
53. Rendall M, Aracil E, Bagavos C, Couet C, DeRose A, DiGiulio P, Lappegård T, Robert-Bobée I, Rønsen M, Smallwood S, Verropoulou G. Increasingly heterogeneous ages at first birth by education in southern European and Anglo-American family-policy regimes: a seven-country comparison by birth cohort. Popul Stud. 2010;64(3):209–27.
54. Adsera A. Vanishing children: from high unemployment to low fertility in developed countries. Am Econ Rev Pap Proc. 2005;95(2):189–93.
55. Cooke A, Mills TA, Lavender T. 'Informed and uninformed decision making'—Women's reasoning, experiences and perceptions with regard to advanced maternal age and delayed childbearing: a meta-synthesis. Int J Nurs Stud. 2010;47(10):1317–29.
56. Gregory E. Ready: why women are embracing the new later motherhood. New York: Basic Books; 2007.
57. Bongaarts J, Sobotka T. A demographic explanation for the recent rise in European fertility. Popul Dev Rev. 2012;38(1):83–120.
58. VID. European Demographic Data Sheet 2016. Vienna Institute of Demography and IIASA/Wittgenstein Centre for Demography and Global Human Capital. 2016. Accessed www.populationeurope.org
59. Leopold T, Skopek J. The delay of grandparenthood: a cohort comparison in East and West Germany. J Marriage Fam. 2015;77(2):441–60.
60. Schmidt L, Sobotka T, Bentzen JG, Nyboe Andersen A. Demographic and medical consequences of the postponement of parenthood. Hum Reprod Update. 2012;18(1):29–43.
61. Goldstein J, Lutz W, Scherbov S. Long-term population decline in Europe: The relative importance of tempo-effects and generational length. Popul Dev Rev. 2003;29(4):699–707.

62. Leridon H, Slama R. The impact of a decline in fecundity and of pregnancy postponement on final number of children and demand for assisted reproduction technology. Hum Reprod. 2008;23(6):1312–9.
63. Te Velde E, Habbema D, Leridon H, Eijkemans M. The effect of postponement of first motherhood on permanent involuntary childlessness and total fertility rate in six European countries since the 1970s. Hum Reprod. 2012;27(4):1179–83.
64. Beemsterboer SN, Homburg R, Gorter NA, Schats R, Hompes PGA, Lambalk CB. The paradox of declining fertility but increasing twinning rates with advancing maternal age. Hum Reprod. 2006;21(6):1531–2.
65. Pison G, Monden C, Smits J. Twinning rates in developed countries: trends and explanations. Popul Dev Rev. 2015;41(4):629–49.
66. Black M, Bhattacharya S. Epidemiology of multiple pregnancy and the effect of assisted conception. Semin Fetal Neonatal Med. 2010;15(6):306–12.
67. Cook JL, Collins J, Buckett W, Racowsky C, Hughes E, Jarvi K. Assisted reproductive technology-related multiple births: Canada in an international context. J Obstet Gynaecol Can. 2011;33(2):159–67.
68. Källén B, Finnström O, Lindam A, Nilsson E, Nygren KG, Olausson PO. Trends in delivery and neonatal outcome after in vitro fertilization in Sweden: data for 25 years. Hum Reprod. 2010;25(4):1026–34.
69. Umstad MP, Hale L, Wang YA, Sullivan EA. Multiple deliveries: The reduced impact of in vitro fertilisation in Australia. Aust N Z J Obstet Gynaecol. 2013;53(2):158–64.
70. Balasch J, Gratacós E. Delayed childbearing: effects on fertility and the outcome of pregnancy. Curr Opin Obstet Gynecol. 2012;24(3):187–93.
71. Bianco A, Stone J, Lynch L, Lapinski R, Berkowitz G, Berkowitz RL. Pregnancy outcome at age 40 and older. Obstet Gynecol. 1996;87(6):917–22.
72. Delbaere I, Verstraelen H, Goetgeluk S, Martens G, De Backer G, Temmerman M. Pregnancy outcome in primiparae of advanced maternal age. Eur J Obstet Gynecol Reprod Biol. 2007;135(1):41–6.
73. Jacobsson B, Ladfors L, Milsom I. Advanced maternal age and adverse perinatal outcome. Obstet Gynecol. 2004;104(4):727–33.
74. Luke B, Brown MB. Contemporary risks of maternal morbidity and adverse outcomes with increasing maternal age and plurality. Fertil Steril. 2007;88(2):283–93.
75. Nybo Andersen AM, Wohlfahrt J, Christens P, Olsen J, Melbye M. Maternal age and fetal loss: population based register linkage study. BMJ. 2000;320(7251):1708–12.
76. de La Rochebrochard E, Thonneau P. Paternal age and maternal age are risk factors for miscarriage; results of a multicentre European study. Hum Reprod. 2002;17(6):1649–56.
77. Abdalla HI, Burton G, Kirkland A, Johnson MR, Leonard T, Brooks AA, Studd JW. Pregnancy: age, pregnancy and miscarriage: uterine versus ovarian factors. Hum Reprod. 1993;8(9):1512–7.
78. Schieve LA, Tatham L, Peterson HB, Toner J, Jeng G. Spontaneous abortion among pregnancies conceived using assisted reproductive technology in the United States. Obstet Gynecol. 2003;101(5, Part 1):959–67.
79. Habbema JDF, Eijkemans MJ, Leridon H, te Velde ER. Realizing a desired family size: when should couples start? Hum Reprod. 2015;30(9):2215–21.
80. Joseph KS, Allen AC, Dodds L, Turner LA, Scott H, Liston R. The perinatal effects of delayed childbearing. Obstet Gynecol. 2005;105(6):1410–8.
81. Voigt M, Briese V, Carstensen M, Wolterdorf F, Hallier E, Straube S. Age-specific preterm birth rates after exclusion of risk factors—an analysis of the German Perinatal Survey. Z Geburtshilfe Neonatol. 2010;214(4):161–6.
82. Heslehurst N, Ells LJ, Simpson H, Batterham A, Wilkinson J, Summerbell CD. Trends in maternal obesity incidence rates, demographic predictors, and health inequalities in 36 821 women over a 15-year period. BJOG Int J Obstet Gynaecol. 2007;114(2):187–94.
83. Luke B, Brown MB, Nugent C, Gonzalez-Quintero VH, Witter FR, Newman RB. Risk factors for adverse outcomes in spontaneous versus assisted conception twin pregnancies. Fertil Steril. 2004;81(2):315–9.

84. Pinborg A. IVF/ICSI twin pregnancies: risks and prevention. Hum Reprod Update. 2005;11: 575–93.
85. Mulder CH. Home-ownership and family formation. J Housing Built Environ. 2006;21(3): 281–98.
86. Mulder CH, Billari FC. Homeownership regimes and low fertility. Hous Stud. 2010;25(4): 527–41.
87. Clark WA. Do women delay family formation in expensive housing markets? Demogr Res. 2012;27(1):1–24.
88. Lino M. Expenditures on children by families, 2013. U.S. Department of Agriculture; 2014. https://www.cnpp.usda.gov/sites/default/files/expenditures_on_children_by_families/crc2013.pdf
89. Björklund A. Does family policy affect fertility? J Popul Econ. 2006;19(1):3–24.
90. Joshi H. Production, reproduction and education: Women, children and work in a British perspective. Popul Dev Rev. 2002;28(3):445–74.
91. Miller AR. The effects of motherhood timing on career path. J Popul Econ. 2011;24(3):1071–100.
92. Taniguchi H. The timing of childbearing and women's wages. J Marriage Fam. 1999;61(6):1008–19.
93. Herr JL. Measuring the effect of the timing of first birth on wages. J Popul Econ. 2016;29(1):39–72.
94. Engelhardt H, Schreyer J. Timing of first birth and well-being in later life. J Fam Res (Zeitschrift für Familienforschung). 2014;26(3):331–46.
95. Goisis A, Sigle-Rushton W. Childbearing postponement and child well-being: a complex and varied relationship? Demography. 2014;51(5):1821–41.
96. Finer LB, Zolna MR. Unintended pregnancy in the United States: incidence and disparities, 2006. Contraception. 2012;84(5):478–85.
97. Mosher WD, Jones J, Abma JC. Intended and unintended births in the United States: 1982–2010. National health statistics reports 55, July 2012; 2012.
98. Musick K, Michelmore K. Change in the stability of marital and cohabiting unions following the birth of a child. Demography. 2015;52(5):1463–85.
99. Hansen K, Hawkes D, Joshi H. The timing of motherhood, mothers' employment and child outcomes. In: Stillwell J, Coast E, Kneale D, editors. Fertility, living arrangements, care and mobility. New York: Springer; 2009. p. 59–70. Chapter 4.
100. Myrskylä M, Margolis R. Happiness: before and after the kids. Demography. 2014;51(5):1843–66.
101. Barclay K, Myrskylä M. Advanced maternal age and offspring outcomes: reproductive aging and counterbalancing period trends. Popul Dev Rev. 2016;42(1):69–94.
102. Grundy E, Kravdal Ø. Reproductive history and mortality in late middle age among Norwegian men and women. Am J Epidemiol. 2008;167(3):271–9.
103. Jaffe D, Kogan L, Manor O, Gielchinsky Y, Dior U, Laufer N. Influence of late-age births on maternal longevity. Ann Epidemiol. 2015;25(6):387–91.
104. Lee RD, Goldstein JR. Rescaling the life cycle. Longevity and proportionality. In: Carey JR, Tuljapurkar S, editors. Life span. Evolutionary, ecological and demographic perspectives. Supplement to Popul Dev Rev. 2003;29:183–207.
105. Mac Dougall K, Beyene Y, Nachtigall RD. 'Inconvenient biology:' advantages and disadvantages of first-time parenting after age 40 using in vitro fertilization. Hum Reprod. 2012;27(4):1058–65.
106. Daly I, Bewley S. Reproductive ageing and conflicting clocks: King Midas' touch. Reprod Biomed Online. 2013;27(6):722–32.
107. Menken J. Age and fertility. How late can you wait? Demography. 1985;22(4):469–83.

Chapter 3
Treatment Options for Age Related Fertility Loss

Panagiotis Drakopoulos and Nikolaos P. Polyzos

Introduction

Age is probably the strongest determinant of treatment success in women seeking fertility advice. Although pregnancy rates after spontaneous conception or assisted reproductive technologies (ART) are relatively good up to the age of 36–37, live birth rates significantly drop with advancing age. Fertility decline, which is associated with the higher oocyte and embryo aneuploidy rate in women of advanced age, is more profound above the age of 40, given that in these patients miscarriage rates exceed 30% [1].

In this chapter we will discuss the treatment options available for women of advanced age in order to overcome the burden associated with age-related fertility loss. In addition, we will present controversial topics related to age fertility decline, as also future perspectives for the management of this difficult group of patients.

P. Drakopoulos
Centre for Reproductive Medicine, Universitair Ziekenhuis Brussel,
Vrije Universiteit Brussel, Brussels, Belgium

N.P. Polyzos (✉)
Service of Reproductive Medicine, Department of Obstetrics, Gynaecology and Reproduction, University Hospital Quirón Dexeus, Barcelona, Spain

Vrije Universiteit Brussel, Brussels, Belgium
e-mail: n.polyzos@gmail.com

© Springer International Publishing Switzerland 2018

D. Stoop (ed.), *Preventing Age Related Fertility Loss*,
DOI 10.1007/978-3-319-14857-1_3

Age Related Fertility Loss

The number of oocytes decreases naturally and progressively though the process of atresia. The fecundity of women decreases gradually with age, with a steep, significant decrease observed after the age of 37 years [2]. This age-related- related decline in fertility is also accompanied by significant increases in the aneuploidy and spontaneous abortion rates [3] (Chap. 1).

Accordingly, declines in oocyte yields and oocyte quality (i.e. 'ovarian aging') are the primary reasons for deteriorating in vitro fertilization (IVF) outcomes with advancing female age, with oocyte quality determining most of embryo quality and embryo quality determining most of pregnancy and live birth chances.

Data recently published by the Human Fertilisation and Embryology Authority (HFEA) outlines the negative correlation between pregnancy rates and female age for the UK's licensed fertility clinics in 2014 [4]. In that year, the analysis of 67,708 cycles of IVF/ICSI demonstrated that pregnancy rates consistently decline with age. In particular, the pregnancy rate per embryo transfer for women of 38–39 was 30.3%, dropping to 21.3% for the age range 40–42, falling again to 11.3% for ages 43–44, reducing to 2.2% for women aged 45 and over (Fig. 3.1)

In conclusion, undoubtedly age is the best predictor of live birth chances and a key component to the understanding of female reproduction.

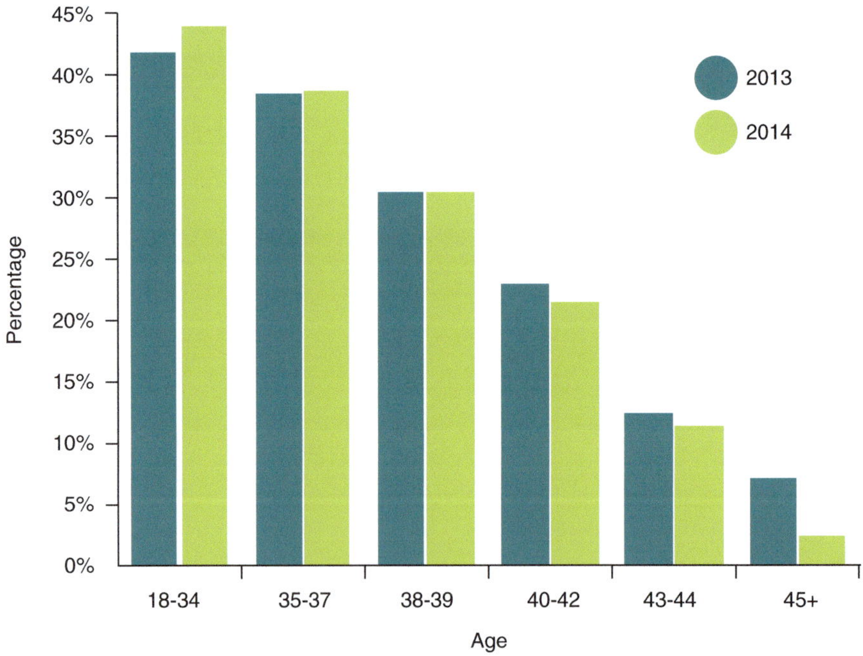

Fig. 3.1 Pregnancy rate (per embryo transfer) for patients receiving IVF treatment using their own fresh eggs, 2013 and 2014. Adapted from Human Fertilisation and Embryology Authority, Fertility Treatment in 2014: Trends and Figures, March 2016

Assisted Reproductive Technologies (ART)

Intrauterine Insemination or In Vitro Fertilization

Infertile counseling is one of the most unpredicted and beautiful part of everyday clinical practice, as it is full of dilemmas. Deciding whether patients should directly be offered IVF or intrauterine insemination (IUI) for the most effective management of their fertility problems is a difficult decision which needs to take into consideration multiple factors, including not only the success rates of each procedure, but also different factors affecting fertility, and obviously the female age.

IUI is often the first choice for most couples in which motile sperm count is reasonable and tubal patency is confirmed.

Female age should always be taken into account when counseling patients, given that current evidence demonstrates disappointing pregnancy rates after IUI (whether or not combined with ovulation induction/stimulation) in women of advanced age, for whom time for conception is critical [5, 6]. The role of age was further emphasized in a large retrospective analysis of 6630 IUI cycles with donor sperm evaluating the cumulative delivery rates of IUI in different age categories [7]. According to the results of the afore mentioned study, it seems that after the fifth IUI cycle, the increase in the delivery rates becomes less apparent and reaches a plateau after the eighth IUI cycle in patients <40 years, whereas the plateau is detected considerably earlier in older patients.

On the other hand, several large series have described IVF outcomes in older patients. On average, live birth rates have been reported to be 8–10% per started cycle in women over the age of 40 [6]. Nevertheless, it should be highlighted that when the data was stratified by yearly age intervals, the results showed a significant decrease in live birth rates with each additional year in age [8].

Consequently, if we consider the age related fertility decline, the accelerated decrease in the ovarian reserve of women of advanced age [9] and the high incidence of embryo aneuploidy which is evident in women above 40 years old, adoption of IVF as a first line treatment may be the best option for this group of infertile patients.

Ovarian Stimulation in Women of Advanced Age

The proportion of women aged 40 years old or over attending IVF/ICSI represents at least 25% of all cycles undertaken in Europe [10].

The 2013 US Society for Assisted Reproductive Technology (SART) data indicated that only 6.6% of fresh nondonor IVF cycles were performed in women above age 42 years, whereas the preliminary 2014 data set suggests that this number increased to 8.4% [11]. This rise in the number of women of advanced age women seeking treatment using their own gametes is mainly due to the improvements of ovarian stimulation over the last decade and the fact that that older patients are no more considered as the "black sheep" for IVF centers, owing to their bad results.

Ovarian stimulation modalities in older women have been poorly studied and most of the available evidence has been derived from studies in poor ovarian responders and young women with unexplained infertility [12].

Based on large observational studies performed in poor responders according to the "Bologna" criteria (which are also certainly fulfilled by a large proportion of women of advanced age), results were consistently low, showing live birth rates of 6% in average, irrespective of the stimulation protocol [Gonadotropin-releasing hormone (GnRH) long, short agonist or GnRH antagonist protocol] and the type of the gonadotropins used [follicle stimulating hormone (FSH) or human menopausal gonadotropin (hMG)] [13–15]. Furthermore, there is sufficient evidence to suggest against the use of high doses above 300 IU of gonadotropins or the supplementation with luteinizing hormone (LH), since no increase will be observed in pregnancy rates [16–18].

On the other hand, inference of evidence on unexplained infertility obtained in young women to the age-related infertility of old women is inappropriate, as the two populations differ significantly. Only one recent randomized trial evaluated this issue in women aged 38–42 years who attempted to seek pregnancy for at least 6 months and whose fertility diagnostic work-up was normal [19]. The patients were randomized into three different arms: (1) two cycles of IUI with clomiphene citrate and then IVF (n = 51), (2) two cycles of IUI with the use of gonadotropins and then IVF (n = 52) and (3) immediate IVF (n = 51). The live birth rate after the first two treatments cycles was higher in the latter group (being 7, 12 and 28% in the three groups, respectively) but the cumulative live birth did not differ (40%, 44% and 41%, respectively).

Natural Cycle IVF and Oocyte Accumulation

Natural Cycle IVF

Natural cycle IVF, which represents a more patient friendly and cost-effective treatment approach has demonstrated very good pregnancy rates in the general infertile population with a cumulative probability of pregnancy up to 46% [20] and this mild approach can be an alternative realistic treatment for many women desiring to avoid ovarian stimulation [20, 21].

Nevertheless, in poor responders, results are disappointing with low live birth rates not exceeding 3% per cycle, regardless of patients' age [22]. Although the afore mentioned study included only poor responders according to the "Bologna" criteria, it seems that even advanced age women who do not fulfill the Bologna criteria, perform as poorly as "Bologna" poor responders [23].

In this regard, there is insufficient evidence to recommend natural cycle IVF as an alternative treatment modality in women of poor prognosis.

Oocyte Accumulation

The idea of oocyte accumulation is based on the assumption that an increase in the number of oocytes retrieved would allow poor responders to be endowed with a normoresponder-like status and yield similar results. Vitrification, as an excellent cryopreservation method could serve for this purpose by creating a large stock of oocytes, accumulated after several stimulation cycles and inseminated in the same time in the future, in an attempt to create more embryos available for transfer.

This hypothesis was tested in a prospective non-randomized study including 724 low responders, showing that live birth rates per patient were significantly higher (30.2% vs. 22.4%) in poor responders choosing the accumulation strategy, suggesting that collection of oocytes could be a reasonable alternative to management of poor prognosis patients [24]. Nevertheless, these finding should be evaluated with skepticism due to the fact that after stratification by age, no significant difference in live birth rates was identified for patients <40 years, whereas a small significant difference existed for older women which represented a small part of the cohort, with only 38 allocated to the accumulation strategy group.

Novel Ovarian Stimulation Protocols

Corifollitropin Alfa

One of the most recently developed molecules developed for ovarian stimulation in women undergoing IVF/ICSI is corifollitropin alfa, a long-acting FSH that has been created by the fusion of the carboxy-terminal arm of the beta subunit of human chorionic gonadotropin (hCG) in the FSH molecule through recombinant technology [25].

Large randomized trials in women with normal ovarian response demonstrated good reproductive outcomes with high pregnancy rates and a potentially higher number of oocytes retrieved compared to recombinant FSH [26, 27].

In order to investigate the efficacy of this new gonadotropin in women with poor ovarian response, preliminary, pilot studies have been conducted in this special infertile population. However, although administration of corifollitropin alfa followed by the administration of hMG in an antagonist protocol may indeed offer benefits in terms of pregnancy rates in women <40 years, results remain low for older women regardless of the protocol or the gonadotropin used [28–30].

Therefore, currently there is no evidence to suggest the use of corifollitropin alpha in older patients, in an attempt to increase their reproductive outcome.

Dual Stimulation

The classic IVF procedure starts with ovarian stimulation in the early follicular phase, in an attempt to retrieve mature oocytes after several days of gonadotropins injections. Luteal phase stimulation has been originally used in case of emergency fertility preservation [31]. The fact that luteal antral follicles may have the same reproductive potential as follicular ones [32], was the trigger to hypothesize that more oocytes and embryos could be harvested if both follicular and luteal stimulation are used in the same menstrual cycle.

The hypothesis of double stimulation was tested in a pilot study including 38 poor responders according to "Bologna" criteria [33]. In summary, the first (follicular) stage of the so-called Shanghai protocol included the administration of a mild stimulation regimen of 150 IU of hMG combined with clomiphene citrate and letrozole, whereas in the second (luteal) stage, a total of 225 hMG IU and letrozole were administered daily from the day of, or the day after the first pick up. All embryos harvested from the two oocyte retrievals were cryopreserved and transferred in subsequent frozen cycles. Although the results of the Shanghai protocol seem promising, as 26 out of 38 patients (68.4%) succeeded in producing 1–6 viable embryos for later use, great caution is needed due the small sample size and the pilot design of the study.

In the same context, Ubaldi et al. [34] performed a prospective non inferiority observational study including 43 patients with reduced ovarian reserve, undergoing follicular and luteal phase stimulation with identical protocols in the same menstrual cycle, in a preimplantation genetic diagnosis for aneuploidy program. The primary outcome was the euploid blastocyst formation rates per metaphase II (MII) oocyte retrieved and the investigators found that both follicular and luteal phase stimulation yielded similar number of euploid blastocysts. Furthermore, luteal phase stimulation contributed significantly to an increase in the cumulative number of available transferrable embryos.

However, it should be highlighted that although these results seem indeed attractive and promising, it's too early to guide clinicians towards the adoption of these approaches and certainly further studies are needed before implementing them to clinical practice.

Preimplanation Genetic Screening

The goal of preimplantation genetic screening (PGS) is the transfer of a euploid embryo aiming at achieving a healthy pregnancy. Although universal application of this technology to all infertile patients undergoing IVF is an issue of debate mainly due to its cost, invasiveness and lack of RCTs of impeccable quality [35], it seems that older women may benefit from PGS [36, 37].

However, it should be highlighted that even if clinical pregnancy and live birth rates appear to be higher in older patients undergoing PGS using advanced techniques of 24-chromosome screening, it seems that that the benefit is merely for those who reach the stage of embryo transfer and have euploid embryos to transfer, as the per cycle advantage in this age group does not persist [36]. Therefore, the application of PGS seems to be of value only for a small subset of poor prognosis patients who are good responders and produce good quality embryos.

Older women should be counseled that several IVF cycles might be required to achieve a single euploid transfer.

Adjuvant Treatments

Growth Hormone

Adjuvant treatment with growth hormone (GH) during ovarian stimulation for IVF/ICSI has been of great interest as an option to improve the outcome in women with poor ovarian response. The rationale for utilizing GH derived from early experimental studies, which demonstrated that GH stimulated the production of insulin-like growth factor (IGF) [38]. Thus, taking into consideration that IGF-1 has been shown to have synergistic effects with FSH on follicular development [39], it may be postulated that GH stimulates ovarian steroidogenesis and follicular development and thus may enhance oocyte quality.

Several small randomized controlled trials have been conducted the last 15 years evaluating the value of adding GH during ovarian stimulation of women with poor ovarian response undergoing IVF/ICSI. However, the sample size of these trials was considerably small, whereas the daily GH dose differed among different trials. A meta-analysis of those randomized trials in 2006 demonstrated that pregnancy rates were significantly higher in the GH group [40], whereas results were similar in an updated meta-analysis in 2010 with an odds ratio (95% CI) 3.28 (1.74–6.20) in favor of GH treatment [41].

Although results from these meta-analyses support the use of GH in poor ovarian response, results should be interpreted with great caution due to the lack of safety data, the small size of the trials included and the limited number of patients enrolled. Furthermore, a recent, not yet published, randomized double blind placebo controlled study of GH administration in poor responders, which was early terminated after 4 years due to poor recruitment, failed to identify any significant in the 131 participants allocated to the randomized arms [42].

Thus, at the moment the evidence is severely "undergrown" in order to recommend routine use in clinical practice.

Androgens

Androgen pre-treatment has probably been one of the most controversial, however widely off-label used treatment options for women with poor ovarian response. According to a survey analysis more than 25% of IVF centers utilize Dehydroepiandrosterone (DHEA) for the treatment of poor ovarian responders (www.ivfworldwide.com).

DHEA is a pre-androgen produced primarily by the adrenal glands with distinct variability in its peripheral conversion to testosterone. Despite the initial enthusiasm derived from the promising results of several cohort and small randomized trials studies using DHEA in poor ovarian responders undergoing IVF/ICSI treatment, recent well-designed RCTs did not find any significant improvement in reproductive outcomes of these women [43].

On the other hand, testosterone, an androgen which directly binds to the androgen receptor may indeed have a role in poor responders. Evidence is derived from studies in primates showing that testosterone stimulates primordial follicle activation and increases the number of growing follicles by increasing IGF-follicular production [44]. It appears that testosterone mainly acts in the early stages of folliculogenesis, by affecting follicular activation and growth [45]. In this regard, long administration of testosterone is mandatory in order to be able to detect a beneficial effect (if any).

Nevertheless, it seems that lessons from ovarian physiology have not been well interpreted by clinical research, as in most of the small available randomized trials, transdermal testosterone in relatively high doses (which could be even detrimental for folliculogenesis) was administered before ovarian stimulation with a duration varying from 5 to 21 days [46, 47].

In conclusion, available literature regarding the use of androgens in women with poor ovarian response (including older patients) is limited. As far as DHEA is concerned, results of randomized trials are robust enough to clearly not recommend its use in an attempt to improve outcomes of ovarian stimulation, whereas results from available randomized trials regarding the use of transdermal testosterone should be evaluated with great caution mainly due to the different doses used and the short duration of administration.

In this context, the results of one of the largest ongoing multicenter double-blind randomized trials (T TRANSPORT study; clinical trials registration number: NCT02418572) in poor responders using a daily dose of 5.5 mg of testosterone which exceeds 60 days of administration, are expected in order to shed more light for the role of androgens in human reproduction and provide final guidance for their use in IVF practice.

In Vitro Activation of Primordial Follicles

The duration of female infertility span depends on the size of the primordial follicle pool and by the rate of its activation and depletion. Activation is the initial and most important step during folliculogenesis, as activated follicles that are not selected for further development will undergo atresia.

However, the molecular mechanisms involved are poorly investigated, although the activation of the PI3K pathway in each individual oocyte may be essential in determining the destiny of the primordial follicle, as demonstrated in genetically modified mice [48]. It seems that short term in vitro activation (IVA) of dormant ovarian follicles after disruption of the Hippo signaling and stimulation of the PI3K pathway allows the generation of a large stock of mature oocytes that could be retrieved and used for IVF in murine [49, 50].

Interestingly, similar patterns have been identified in human oocytes. In fact, it was recently shown that ovarian cryopreservation, fragmentation and IVA drug treatment, followed by auto-transplantation in a small number of patients with primary ovarian insufficiency, could lead to the generation of functional mature oocytes for infertility treatment [51].

If these preliminary results are replicated in further larger studies including patients of advanced age or women with diminished ovarian reserve, news horizons could be opened up.

Oocyte Donation

Oocyte donation was initially developed as a therapy for young women with premature ovarian failure, rather than as a means of overcoming the age-related decline in fertility. However, age-related infertility is now one of the most common reasons to use oocyte donation, especially in women over 40 years of age. Cumulative pregnancy rates after 4 cycles of embryo transfer have been reported to be as high as 90%, irrespective of recipient's age [52].

However, obstetrical and neonatal complications related to advanced maternal age should not be overlooked, especially given the increasing demand for the availability of oocyte donors. A recent meta-analysis reported elevated risks of hypertensive disorders of pregnancy, preeclampsia, low birth weight, preterm birth, cesarean section and postpartum haemorrhage in pregnancies achieved after oocyte donation versus IVF or spontaneously conceived pregnancies [53].

Lastly, it should be highlighted that differences in the donation programs exist from country to country and raise ethical and legal issues such as financial compensation of the donors, their anonymity and the waiting time of enrolled patients in the donation program.

Key Messages

1. The age related decline in fertility is accompanied by significant increases in the aneuploidy and spontaneous abortion rates.
2. Adoption of IVF as a first line treatment may be the best option in women above 40 years old.
3. There is insufficient evidence to recommend natural cycle IVF, oocyte accumulation or novel ovarian stimulation protocols including dual stimulation as alternative treatment modalities in women of poor prognosis.
4. Testosterone pre-treatment in women with poor ovarian response may be an option, but more evidence derived by well-designed randomized studies is needed.
5. Oocyte donation is an excellent treatment option with high success rates, although obstetrical and neonatal complications related to advanced maternal age should be taken into account.

References

1. Farr SL, Schieve LA, Jamieson DJ. Pregnancy loss among pregnancies conceived through assisted reproductive technology, United States, 1999–2002. Am J Epidemiol. 2007;165(12):1380–8.
2. American College of O, Gynecologists Committee on Gynecologic P, Practice C. Female age-related fertility decline. Committee Opinion No. 589. Fertil Steril. 2014;101(3):633–4.
3. Balasch J, Gratacos E. Delayed childbearing: effects on fertility and the outcome of pregnancy. Curr Opin Obstet Gynecol. 2012;24(3):187–93.
4. (HFEA) HFaEA. Fertility treatment in 2014: Trends and figures. 2016. Available at www.hfea.gov.uk.
5. Wiser A, Shalom-Paz E, Reinblatt SL, Son WY, Das M, Tulandi T, et al. Ovarian stimulation and intrauterine insemination in women aged 40 years or more. Reprod Biomed Online. 2012;24(2):170–3.
6. Armstrong S, Akande V. What is the best treatment option for infertile women aged 40 and over? J Assist Reprod Genet. 2013;30(5):667–71.
7. De Brucker M, Haentjens P, Evenepoel J, Devroey P, Collins J, Tournaye H. Cumulative delivery rates in different age groups after artificial insemination with donor sperm. Hum Reprod. 2009;24(8):1891–9.
8. Tsafrir A, Simon A, Margalioth EJ, Laufer N. What should be the first-line treatment for unexplained infertility in women over 40 years of age - ovulation induction and IUI, or IVF? Reprod Biomed Online. 2009;19(Suppl 4):4334.
9. Iliodromiti S, Iglesias Sanchez C, Messow CM, Cruz M, Garcia Velasco J, Nelson SM. Excessive age-related decline in functional ovarian reserve in infertile women: prospective cohort of 15,500 women. J Clin Endocrinol Metab. 2016;101(9):3548–54.
10. Andersen AN, Goossens V, Ferraretti AP, Bhattacharya S, Felberbaum R, de Mouzon J, et al. Assisted reproductive technology in Europe, 2004: results generated from European registers by ESHRE. Hum Reprod. 2008;23(4):756–71.
11. Gleicher N, Kushnir VA, Albertini DF, Barad DH. Improvements in IVF in women of advanced age. J Endocrinol. 2016;230(1):F1–6.
12. Somigliana E, Paffoni A, Busnelli A, Filippi F, Pagliardini L, Vigano P, et al. Age-related infertility and unexplained infertility: an intricate clinical dilemma. Hum Reprod. 2016;31(7):1390–6.
13. Polyzos NP, Nwoye M, Corona R, Blockeel C, Stoop D, Haentjens P, et al. Live birth rates in Bologna poor responders treated with ovarian stimulation for IVF/ICSI. Reprod Biomed Online. 2014;28(4):469–74.
14. Busnelli A, Papaleo E, Del Prato D, La Vecchia I, Iachini E, Paffoni A, et al. A retrospective evaluation of prognosis and cost-effectiveness of IVF in poor responders according to the Bologna criteria. Hum Reprod. 2015;30(2):315–22.
15. La Marca A, Grisendi V, Giulini S, Sighinolfi G, Tirelli A, Argento C, et al. Live birth rates in the different combinations of the Bologna criteria poor ovarian responders: a validation study. J Assist Reprod Genet. 2015;32(6):931–7.
16. Berkkanoglu M, Isikoglu M, Aydin D, Ozgur K. Clinical effects of ovulation induction with recombinant follicle-stimulating hormone supplemented with recombinant luteinizing hormone or low-dose recombinant human chorionic gonadotropin in the midfollicular phase in microdose cycles in poor responders. Fertil Steril. 2007;88(3):665–9.
17. Lefebvre J, Antaki R, Kadoch IJ, Dean NL, Sylvestre C, Bissonnette F, et al. 450 IU versus 600 IU gonadotropin for controlled ovarian stimulation in poor responders: a randomized controlled trial. Fertil Steril. 2015;104(6):1419–25.
18. Kolibianakis EM, Kalogeropoulou L, Griesinger G, Papanikolaou EG, Papadimas J, Bontis J, et al. Among patients treated with FSH and GnRH analogues for in vitro fertilization, is the

addition of recombinant LH associated with the probability of live birth? A systematic review and meta-analysis. Hum Reprod Update. 2007;13(5):445–52.
19. Goldman MB, Thornton KL, Ryley D, Alper MM, Fung JL, Hornstein MD, et al. A randomized clinical trial to determine optimal infertility treatment in older couples: the Forty and Over Treatment Trial (FORT-T). Fertil Steril. 2014;101(6):1574–81. e1–2
20. Nargund G, Waterstone J, Bland J, Philips Z, Parsons J, Campbell S. Cumulative conception and live birth rates in natural (unstimulated) IVF cycles. Hum Reprod. 2001;16(2):259–62.
21. Pelinck MJ, Vogel NE, Hoek A, Simons AH, Arts EG, Mochtar MH, et al. Cumulative pregnancy rates after three cycles of minimal stimulation IVF and results according to subfertility diagnosis: a multicentre cohort study. Hum Reprod. 2006;21(9):2375–83.
22. Polyzos NP, Blockeel C, Verpoest W, De Vos M, Stoop D, Vloeberghs V, et al. Live birth rates following natural cycle IVF in women with poor ovarian response according to the Bologna criteria. Hum Reprod. 2012;27(12):3481–6.
23. Schimberni M, Morgia F, Colabianchi J, Giallonardo A, Piscitelli C, Giannini P, et al. Natural-cycle in vitro fertilization in poor responder patients: a survey of 500 consecutive cycles. Fertil Steril. 2009;92(4):1297–301.
24. Cobo A, Garrido N, Crespo J, Jose R, Pellicer A. Accumulation of oocytes: a new strategy for managing low-responder patients. Reprod Biomed Online. 2012;24(4):424–32.
25. Fares FA, Suganuma N, Nishimori K, LaPolt PS, Hsueh AJ, Boime I. Design of a long-acting follitropin agonist by fusing the C-terminal sequence of the chorionic gonadotropin beta subunit to the follitropin beta subunit. Proc Natl Acad Sci U S A. 1992;89(10):4304–8.
26. Corifollitropin alfa Ensure Study G. Corifollitropin alfa for ovarian stimulation in IVF: a randomized trial in lower-body-weight women. Reprod Biomed Online. 2010;21(1):66–76.
27. Devroey P, Boostanfar R, Koper NP, Mannaerts BM, Ijzerman-Boon PC, Fauser BC, et al. A double-blind, non-inferiority RCT comparing corifollitropin alfa and recombinant FSH during the first seven days of ovarian stimulation using a GnRH antagonist protocol. Hum Reprod. 2009;24(12):3063–72.
28. Polyzos NP, Devos M, Humaidan P, Stoop D, Ortega-Hrepich C, Devroey P, et al. Corifollitropin alfa followed by rFSH in a GnRH antagonist protocol for poor ovarian responder patients: an observational pilot study. Fertil Steril. 2013;99(2):422–6.
29. Polyzos NP, Corona R, Van De Vijver A, Blockeel C, Drakopoulos P, Vloeberghs V, et al. Corifollitropin alfa followed by hpHMG in GnRH agonist protocols. Two prospective feasibility studies in poor ovarian responders. Gynecol Endocrinol. 2015;31(11):885–90.
30. Polyzos NP, De Vos M, Corona R, Vloeberghs V, Ortega-Hrepich C, Stoop D, et al. Addition of highly purified HMG after corifollitropin alfa in antagonist-treated poor ovarian responders: a pilot study. Hum Reprod. 2013;28(5):1254–60.
31. von Wolff M, Thaler CJ, Frambach T, Zeeb C, Lawrenz B, Popovici RM, et al. Ovarian stimulation to cryopreserve fertilized oocytes in cancer patients can be started in the luteal phase. Fertil Steril. 2009;92(4):1360–5.
32. Baerwald AR, Adams GP, Pierson RA. A new model for ovarian follicular development during the human menstrual cycle. Fertil Steril. 2003;80(1):116–22.
33. Kuang Y, Chen Q, Hong Q, Lyu Q, Ai A, Fu Y, et al. Double stimulations during the follicular and luteal phases of poor responders in IVF/ICSI programmes (Shanghai protocol). Reprod Biomed Online. 2014;29(6):684–91.
34. Ubaldi FM, Capalbo A, Vaiarelli A, Cimadomo D, Colamaria S, Alviggi C, et al. Follicular versus luteal phase ovarian stimulation during the same menstrual cycle (DuoStim) in a reduced ovarian reserve population results in a similar euploid blastocyst formation rate: new insight in ovarian reserve exploitation. Fertil Steril. 2016;105(6):1488–95. e1
35. Mastenbroek S, Repping S. Preimplantation genetic screening: back to the future. Hum Reprod. 2014;29(9):1846–50.
36. Kang HJ, Melnick AP, Stewart JD, Xu K, Rosenwaks Z. Preimplantation genetic screening: who benefits? Fertil Steril. 2016;106(3):597–602.

37. Harton GL, Munne S, Surrey M, Grifo J, Kaplan B, McCulloh DH, et al. Diminished effect of maternal age on implantation after preimplantation genetic diagnosis with array comparative genomic hybridization. Fertil Steril. 2013;100(6):1695–703.
38. Doldi N, Bassan M, Bonzi V, Ferrari A. Effects of growth hormone and growth hormone-releasing hormone on steroid synthesis in cultured human luteinizing granulosa cells. Gynecol Endocrinol. 1996;10(2):101–8.
39. Adashi EY, Rohan RM. Intraovarian regulation: peptidergic signaling systems. Trends Endocrinol Metab. 1992;3(7):243–8.
40. Kolibianakis EM, Venetis CA, Diedrich K, Tarlatzis BC, Griesinger G. Addition of growth hormone to gonadotrophins in ovarian stimulation of poor responders treated by in-vitro fertilization: a systematic review and meta-analysis. Hum Reprod Update. 2009;15(6):613–22.
41. Duffy JM, Ahmad G, Mohiyiddeen L, Nardo LG, Watson A. Growth hormone for in vitro fertilization. Cochrane Database Syst Rev. 2010; (1):CD000099.
42. Investigators NReatL. A randomised double blind placebo controlled study of recombinant human growth hormone (r-HGH) on live birth rates in women who are poor responders. In: 32nd annual meeting of the European Society of Human Reproduction and Embryology. Helsinki, Finland: Oxford University Press; 2016.
43. Yeung TW, Chai J, Li RH, Lee VC, Ho PC, Ng EH. A randomized, controlled, pilot trial on the effect of dehydroepiandrosterone on ovarian response markers, ovarian response, and in vitro fertilization outcomes in poor responders. Fertil Steril. 2014;102(1):108–15. e1
44. Weil S, Vendola K, Zhou J, Bondy CA. Androgen and follicle-stimulating hormone interactions in primate ovarian follicle development. J Clin Endocrinol Metab. 1999;84(8):2951–6.
45. Walters KA. Role of androgens in normal and pathological ovarian function. Reproduction. 2015;149(4):R193–218.
46. Polyzos NP, Davis SR, Drakopoulos P, Humaidan P, De Geyter C, Vega AG, et al. Testosterone for poor ovarian responders: lessons from ovarian physiology. Reprod Sci. 2016 Aug 3. pii: 1933719116660849. [Epub ahead of print].
47. Gonzalez-Comadran M, Duran M, Sola I, Fabregues F, Carreras R, Checa MA. Effects of transdermal testosterone in poor responders undergoing IVF: systematic review and meta-analysis. Reprod Biomed Online. 2012;25(5):450–9.
48. Reddy P, Liu L, Adhikari D, Jagarlamudi K, Rajareddy S, Shen Y, et al. Oocyte-specific deletion of Pten causes premature activation of the primordial follicle pool. Science. 2008;319(5863):611–3.
49. Li J, Kawamura K, Cheng Y, Liu S, Klein C, Liu S, et al. Activation of dormant ovarian follicles to generate mature eggs. Proc Natl Acad Sci U S A. 2010;107(22):10280–4.
50. Kawamura K, Cheng Y, Suzuki N, Deguchi M, Sato Y, Takae S, et al. Hippo signaling disruption and Akt stimulation of ovarian follicles for infertility treatment. Proc Natl Acad Sci U S A. 2013;110(43):17474–9.
51. Suzuki N, Yoshioka N, Takae S, Sugishita Y, Tamura M, Hashimoto S, et al. Successful fertility preservation following ovarian tissue vitrification in patients with primary ovarian insufficiency. Hum Reprod. 2015;30(3):608–15.
52. Remohi J, Gartner B, Gallardo E, Yalil S, Simon C, Pellicer A. Pregnancy and birth rates after oocyte donation. Fertil Steril. 1997;67(4):717–23.
53. Storgaard M, Loft A, Bergh C, Wennerholm UB, Soderstrom-Anttila V, Romundstad LB, et al. Obstetric and neonatal complications in pregnancies conceived after oocyte donation—a systematic review and meta-analysis. BJOG. 2017;124:561–72.

Chapter 4
Preliminary Assessment Prior to Oocyte Cryopreservation

O. Rustamov and S.K. Sunkara

Introduction

It has been estimated that around 90% of primordial follicles are lost by the age of 30 years, which is an average age of women starting family in most western countries [1, 2]. This suggests most women start trying to conceive in a state of depleted ovarian reserve; consequently, in some this leads to infertility and childlessness. Therefore, availability of Fertility Preservation Services is emerging as a basic health necessity for some women. Owing to recent advances in techniques for oocyte vitrification an option of effective fertility preservation, long before women have made reproductive decisions, has become available. However due to a range of factors which include lack of societal acceptance, inadequate awareness among patients as well as health care professionals, the economic cost and the organisational challenges, Fertility Preservation services are not readily accessible.

In principal, care pathway of Oocyte Cryopreservation can be divided into four distinct stages: (1) preliminary assessment, (2) controlled ovarian stimulation, (3) oocyte recovery and cryopreservation and (4) post treatment counselling. Preliminary assessment is of paramount importance, given that the effectiveness of subsequent stages of the management are largely determined by this evaluation. In addition, pre-treatment consultation provides an excellent opportunity to develop an understanding with the patient which can be invaluable in care of patients undergoing a potentially stressful treatment.

In this chapter, the interventions for the preliminary assessment prior to oocyte cryopreservation has been discussed in a stepwise manner reflecting the patient

O. Rustamov (✉)
Aberdeen Centre of Reproductive Medicine, University of Aberdeen, Aberdeen, UK
e-mail: oybek_rustamov@yahoo.co.uk

S.K. Sunkara
Queen's Hospital, Barking Havering and Redbridge University Hospitals, Essex, UK

© Springer International Publishing Switzerland 2018

D. Stoop (ed.), *Preventing Age Related Fertility Loss*,
DOI 10.1007/978-3-319-14857-1_4

journey in real clinical conditions. The merit of each intervention has been appraised in the light of availability of the scientific evidence on its effectiveness. More importantly the quality of the evidence itself has been subjected to a robust interrogation, providing in depth analysis of the whole process.

A thorough preliminary assessment should include following stages: (1) history taking; (2) physical examination, (3) pelvic ultrasound scanning, (4) assessment of ovarian reserve, (5) genetic testing and (6) pre-treatment counselling.

History Taking

It is important to note, that the choice of treatment interventions may vary according to patient characteristics and expectations. Therefore, the reason for requesting oocyte cryopreservation and the outcome patient expects from the treatment ought to be established. For instance, the treatment pathway of a young patient wishing fertility preservation prior to achieving career goals may differ to that of someone with a family history of premature ovarian insufficiency. Consequently, achieving an understanding of the reason behind the need for oocyte cryopreservation is of importance.

History on general health should be established to evaluate safety of ovarian stimulation and oocyte recovery procedures as well as implications of a future pregnancy on patient's health. Reproductive history includes, age at menarche, duration of menstrual cycles, the date of last menstrual cycle, use of contraceptives, previous gynaecological pathologies and previous obstetric history. As part of a social history clinicians may seek if the patient is in a stable relationship, patient's plans for future fertility and if there are any relevant social issues that may affect future plans for starting a family.

Importantly, by way of directed history taking, risk factors for loss of ovarian reserve should be ascertained. Ovarian reserve is determined by assembly of primordial follicles during embryonic and fetal period as well as subsequent rate of loss of oocytes, both of which appear to be largely under the influence of genetic, environmental, life style and medical factors [3, 4]. Studies have demonstrated that there is a significant association between maternal age at menopause and the ovarian reserve of a woman [5]. Therefore, establishing this and reproductive history of the patient's mother and sisters provide important insight into a genetic predisposition of the patient to premature ovarian insufficiency (POI). The effect of environmental factors on ovarian reserve is not fully explored. However, there is convincing evidence on detrimental impact of certain agents such as radiation and gonadotoxic chemicals. Similarly, some life style factors such as smoking affect the patient's ovarian reserve as well as reproductive performance in general. The role of certain medical factors on the ovarian reserve have been studied in depth which can largely be divided into three broad medical modalities: Radiotherapy, Chemotherapy and Surgical Intervention on ovaries. Although all these interventions appear to have detrimental effect on ovarian reserve, there is considerable variation between the effect of individual treatments. For instance, some chemotherapeutic agents display a potent gonadotoxic effect whilst others may result in mild and temporary cessation of the patient's reproductive performance [6]. Similarly, the duration as well as dose of chemotherapeutic agents are also recognised determinants of subsequent ovarian reserve. Therefore obtaining detailed history on exposure to Genetic, Environmental, Life Style and Medical Factors for accelerated loss of ovarian reserve provides important insight into the patient's current and future fertility, which is instrumental in counselling an individual patient with regards to their fertility preservation.

In contrast, the role of other factors on the ovarian reserve is less understood. For instance, findings of studies on the role of ethnicity with ovarian reserve is conflicting. Some studies reported significant association between patient's ethnicity and AMH levels [4, 7] whilst other did not find any correlation of AMH with ethnicity [8]. Similarly, a recent study which compared all three main markers (AMH, AFC, FSH) in a large cohort of infertile women (n = 2946) found that the effect of ethnicity on the markers of ovarian reserve was weak; suggesting prediction of the decline of ovarian reserve of individual patients on the basis of ethnicity is not feasible [9].

Physical Examination

Basic anthropometric measurements such as height, weight and body mass index allows to evaluate overall wellbeing of the patient. However, the role of BMI in understanding of individual patient's ovarian reserve is less understood. Whilst some report that higher body weight is associated with lower AMH [7, 10, 11], other studies found obese women have significantly higher AMH, AFC and lower FSH measurements levels suggesting direct correlation between weight and ovarian reserve [12].

Ultrasound

Pelvic pathology may have significant impact on both oocyte cryopreservation cycle and future fertility treatment. Therefore presence of uterine, tubal and ovarian pathologies should be ruled out prior to oocyte cryopreservation treatment cycle. Consequently, ultrasound scanning should be utilised as a tool for screening. In addition ultrasound scan offers one of the best tools for assessment of ovarian reserve, antral follicle count (AFC), which has a number of advantages compared to that of other markers of ovarian reserve which as discussed below.

Assessment of Ovarian Reserve

The biological ovarian reserve is defined as the number of primordial and growing follicles left in the ovary at any given time and therefore, establishment of a true biological ovarian reserve is clearly not feasible in clinical setting. However, ovarian reserve can be estimated using various biomarkers, such as Chronological Age, Follicle stimulating hormone (FSH), Anti-Mullerian Hormone (AMH) and Antral Follicle Count (AFC). Although these markers provide best available representation of patient's ovarian reserve, it is important to appreciate the strengths and the limitations of these markers so that they are interpreted within the context of overall characteristics of the tests rather than in absolute numbers. Therefore in order to provide in depth understanding; we first provide a brief review of the biology of ovarian reserve, then discuss technical performance of the tests in light of latest available evidence.

Ovarian Reserve

An ovarian reserve is determined by the size of the oocyte pool at birth and the decline in the oocyte number thereafter. Both of these processes are largely under the influence of genetic factors although environmental and life style factors appear to play a role [13, 4]. Folliculogenesis in women of reproductive age consists of two stages (a) the initial non-cyclical recruitment of primordial follicles leading to the formation of primary and pre-antral follicles and (b) the cyclical development of antral follicles with a subsequent selection of a single dominant follicle (Fig. 4.1). The mechanism of the initial recruitment of the oocytes is not well understood, but it is clear that the process is independent of the influence of the pituitary gonadotrophins and appears to be governed by the genetically pre-programmed interaction of

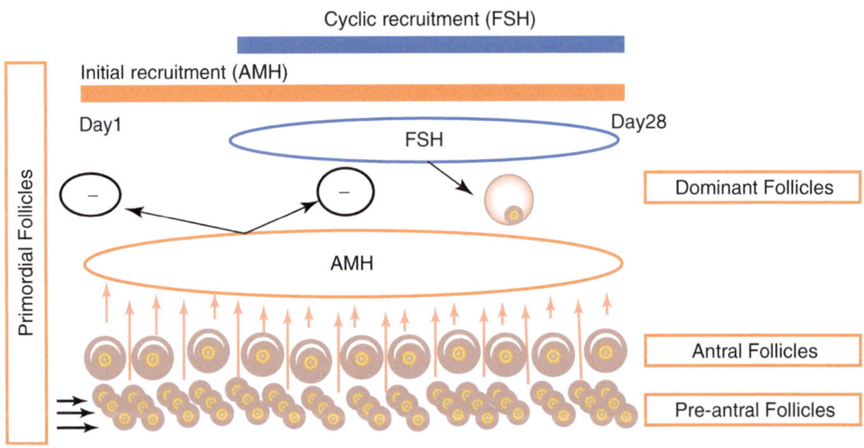

Fig. 4.1 Initial and cyclic recruitment of oocytes: the role of AMH and FSH

the oocyte with local growth factors, the most important of which appears to be anti-Müllerian hormone, and cytokines [3]. Anti-Müllerian hormone appears to be the main regulator of the size of the primordial follicle pool by its inhibitory effect on the recruitment of the primordial follicles [14]. The cyclical phase of development of oocytes is characterised by the transformation of secondary follicles into antral follicles and subsequent growth of the antral follicles into pre-ovulatory stages. In general, the process of cyclic recruitment starts from puberty under the influence of rising levels of pituitary follicular stimulating hormone (FSH). Interestingly, in addition to its inhibitory effect to the resting follicles, AMH also suppresses the development of the growing follicles and it appears that AMH inhibits FSH-induced follicle growth by reducing the sensitivity of growing follicles to FSH [15]. Thus AMH and FSH play a central role in recruitment and growth of follicles which is underpinned by the state of ovarian reserve at given time that is largely determined by the woman's age. Consequently measurement of these parameters, namely AMH, FSH, follicle count (AFC) and age, provides a window into the state of ovarian activity as well as overall reserve of the ovaries in women.

Chronological Age

Owing to the biological age-related decline of the quantity, and arguably the quality, of oocytes the chronological age can be used as a marker of ovarian reserve. Studies have demonstrated that ovarian reserve [2, 16], natural fecundity and outcomes of ART [17, 18] decline significantly from age of 35 when it is believed the ovarian reserve undergoes accelerated decline. Although there is a strong association between chronological age and reduction in fertility, evidently there is a significant variation in age-related ovarian reserve indicating chronological age alone may not be sufficient to estimate the individual woman's ovarian reserve reliably [19].

Basal FSH

Basal FSH was one of the first endocrine markers introduced in assessment of fertility and is still utilised in many fertility clinics, albeit in conjunction with other markers which are considered more reliable. Secretion of FSH is largely governed by the negative feedback effect of steroid hormones, primarily oestradiol, and inhibins which are expressed in granulosa cells of growing ovarian follicles. Consequently, decreased or diminished recruitment of ovarian follicles is associated increased serum FSH measurements and high, particularly very high basal FSH reading is considered as a good marker of very low or diminished ovarian reserve [20]. However, unlike some other markers, FSH measurements do not appear to have discriminatory power for categorisation of patients to various bands of ovarian reserve. Given between-patient variability FSH measurement (CV 30%) is similar to its within-patient variability (27%), stratification of patients to various ranges of ovarian reserve does not appear to be feasible [21]. Indeed, a systematic review of

37 studies on the prediction of poor response and non-pregnancy in IVF cycle has concluded that, basal FSH is an adequate test at very high threshold levels and therefore has limited value in modern ART programs [19].

Antral Follicle Count

Basal antral follicle count estimation involves ultrasound assessment of ovaries between 2nd and 4th day of menstrual period and counting "follicles", which corresponds to antral stage of folliculogenesis [22]. The test provides direct quantitative assessment of growing follicles and is known as one of the most reliable markers of ovarian reserve. AFC measurement has been reported as having a similar sensitivity and specificity to AMH in prediction of poor and excessive ovarian response in IVF cycles [19, 23]. Given AFC measurement is available instantly and allows patients to be counseled immediately, the test eliminates the need for an additional patient visit prior to IVF cycle. However, AFC is normally performed only in the early follicular phase of the menstrual cycle, given most published data on measurement of AFC are based on studies that assessed antral follicles during this stage of the cycle [22]. Interestingly, some studies suggest that variability of AFC during menstrual cycle is small, particularly when follicles between 2 and 6 mm are counted, and therefore assessment of AFC without account for the day of menstrual cycle may be feasible.

One of the main drawbacks of AFC is that the cut off levels for size of counted follicles remains to be standardised [22]. Initially, follicles of 2–10 mm were introduced as the range for AFC and many studies were based on this cut off. Later, counting follicles of 2–6 mm was reported to provide most accurate assessment of ovarian reserve [24, 25] and therefore some newer studies are based on AFC measurements that used this criterion. Consequently, direct comparison of the outcomes of various studies on assessment of AFC requires careful analysis.

Similar to other markers of ovarian reserve (Table 4.1), AFC appears to display significant variability between measurements in same patient [26]. The study that evaluated the measurement AFC (n = 4059) in a large cohort of patient (n = 2362)

Table 4.1 Within- and—between patient variability of AFC, FSH, AMH (Gen II and DSL assays) measurement

	AFC		FSH		AHM (Gen II assay)[a]		AHM (DSL assay)	
Comparsion	Mean (SD)	CV (%)	Mean (SD)	CV (%)	Mean (SD)	CV (%)	Mean (SD)	CV (%)
Between patients	13.9 (6.3)	35	7.4 (2.2)	30	11.2	126	12.7 (12.0)	94
Within-patient		30		27		59		28
Within-sample		ND		6		3.57		4.8

Note: Data on FSH, AFC and AMH (Gen II and DSL assays) are based on population of the same centre [21, 27]

AMH measured in pmol/L, FSH in IU/L, *CV* coefficient of variation, *ND* not determined

[a]Unmodified original Gen II assay (Data collection: 17.11.2010–25.10.2011)

found that within-patient variation of AFC (CV 30%) was similar to that of between patient variation (CV 35%) suggesting that categorisation of the patients into various groups of ovarian reserve on the basis of AFC may not be as reliable as previously thought.

Anti-Müllerian Hormone

In the female, anti-Müllerian hormone (AMH), produced by granulosa cells of preantral and early antral ovarian follicles, regulates oocyte recruitment and folliculogenesis [14]. It can assess ovarian reserve and guide gonadotropin stimulation in assisted reproduction technology [28]. AMH is also used as a granulosa cell tumor marker, a tool for evaluation of ovarian reserve after chemotherapy [29], and to predict age at menopause [30, 31].

AMH immunoassays, first developed by Hudson et al. [32] in 1990, were introduced commercially by Diagnostic Systems Laboratories (DSL) and Immunotech (IOT). These assays were integrated into a second-generation AMH assay (Gen II) by Beckman-Coulter, but studies suggested that this assay exhibited clinically important, within-patient, sample variability [21, 27]. Beckman Coulter confirmed this with a field safety notice (FSN 20434-3) and withdrew the assay kits from use. Subsequently, third generation AMH assays were introduced which include: (1) modified method of Gen II ELISA by Beckman Coulter, (2) Pico AMH Ansh Labs, (3) Ultrasensitive Ansh Labs, (4) Automatic test by Roche ELECSYS and (5) automated verison of Beckman Coulter Gen II ELISA. Important to underline, all above AMH assay tests may share certain common properties due to the fact they most utilise same antibody and/or calibrated against each other. Therefore, they may have common strengths and, more worryingly, possibly same issues. Therefore, there is a clear need for an international reference standard for AMH and for robust independent evaluation of commercial assays in routine clinical samples with well-defined sample handling and processing protocols. Meanwhile, previous issues of sample instability and lack of reliable inter-assay comparability data should be taken into account in the interpretation of available research evidence and the application of AMH measurement in clinical practice.

Genetic Testing

As previously discussed both formation as well as decline of ovarian reserve is largely determined genetically and therefore extremes of poor ovarian reserve such as Premature Ovarian Insufficiency (POI) and Early menopause have genetic origin [33]. Premature ovarian insufficiency may present as a feature of certain genetic syndromes, such as galactosemia and blepharophimosis-ptosis-epicanthus produced by mutations *in FOXL2* gene that can be diagnosed by their non-ovarian phenotype. However, chromosomal abnormalities, mosaic of sex chromosome abnormalities, premutation alleles of FMR1 and other rare mutations are associated to primary premature ovarian failure without other phenotypic features [33]. When premature ovarian insufficiency is suspected, appropriate genetic testing, including a referral to a clinical geneticist is recommended.

Patients concerned about their risk of premature ovarian insufficiency, should be referred to genetic counselling. Pre-symptomatic or carrier genetic testing will depend on family history, patient's medical history and their desire for genetic testing. The most relevant investigations are karyotyping and allele size in FMR1 gene. Analysis of repeats in *FMR1* gene is recommended as preconception or prenatal carrier screening in women with a family history of X-fragile, non-diagnosed mental retardation, developmental delay, autism or ovarian insufficiency [34]. A screening of *FMR1* in a large group (n = 2300) women found a frequency of 1.7% for premutation and 0.61% for full mutation in US [35]. These findings suggest that if women interested in preconceptional fragile X carrier screening, they should be offered the test irrespective of presence of any family history of the condition [34]. In addition, expanded carrier screening including analysis of frequent mutations in more than 100 genetics conditions can be considered in line with the recommendations of American Genetics as well as American Obstetrics and Fetal Medicine Societies [36] and supported by European Society of Human Genetics [37]. Thus, genetic testing in patients undergoing fertility preservation for ovarian ageing is determined by a family history of premature ovarian insufficiency, symptoms of genetic traits associated with premature loss of ovarian reserve and findings of assessment of ovarian reserve.

Pre-treatment Counselling

Once full assessment has taken place, patient should have an opportunity to have individualized pre-treatment counselling. This should include discussion of clinical effectiveness, cost, limitations and logistics of oocyte preservation. Patients should be provided information leaflets which is written in plain language in the format accessible to patients.

Key Message

1. Given the clinical and laboratory advances, demand for oocyte cryopreservation for both medical and social reasons is on the rise in recent times.
2. Counselling should be considered a key priority to enable women in making informed decisions regarding fertility preservation.
3. Clinicians should be aware of the importance of detailed clinical assessment.
4. Particular attention should be given to the assessment of the ovarian reserve.
5. Knowledge of the biological, hormonal and ultrasound markers of ovarian reserve and their predictive ability is vital to the assessment and counselling of women undertaking fertility/oocyte cryopreservation.

References

1. Live births in England and Wales by characteristics of mother. Office of National Statistics. 2012.
2. Wallace WH, Kelsey TW. Human ovarian reserve from conception to the menopause. PLoS One. 2010;5(1):e8772.
3. McGee EA, Hsueh AJ. Initial and cyclic recruitment of ovarian follicles. Endocr Rev. 2000;21(2): 200–14.
4. Schuh-Huerta SM, Johnson NA, Rosen MP, Sternfeld B, Cedars MI, Reijo Pera RA. Genetic variants and environmental factors associated with hormonal markers of ovarian reserve in Caucasian and African American women. Hum Reprod. 2012;27:594–608.
5. Morris DH, Jones ME, Schoemaker MJ, Ashworth A, Swerdlow AJ. Familial concordance for age at natural menopause: results from the Breakthrough Generations Study. Menopause. 2011;18:956–61.
6. Biasoli I, Falorio S, Luminari S, Spector N, Federico M. Fertility in female survivors of Hodgkin's lymphoma. Rev Bras Hematol Hemoter. 2012;34(1):48–53. doi:10.5581/1516-8484.20120014.
7. Seifer DB, Golub ET, Lambert-Messerlian G, Benning L, Anastos K, Watts H, Cohen MH, Karim R, Young MA, Minkoff H, and Greenblatt RM. Variations in serum Mullerian inhibiting substance between white, black and Hispanic women. Fertil Steril. 2009;92(5):1674–8.
8. Freeman EW, Gracia CR, Sammel MD, Lin H, Lim LC, Strauss JF III. Association of anti-mullerian hormone levels with obesity in late reproductive-age women. Fertil Steril. 2007;87:101–6.
9. Krishnan M, Rustamov O, Mathur R, Roberts S, Fitzgerald C. The effect of the ethnicity on the ovarian reserve. British Fertility Society Annual Meeting; 2014.
10. Sahmay S, Usta T, Erel CT, Imamoğlu M, Kuuk M, Atakul N, Seyisoğlu H. Is there any correlation between amh and obesity in premenopausal women? Arch Gynecol Obstet. 2012;286(3): 661–5.
11. Skałba P Cygal A, Madej P, Dabkowska-Huc A, Sikora J, Martirosian G, Romanik M, Olszanecka-Glinianowicz M. Is the plasma anti-Mullerian hormone (AMH) level associated with body weight and metabolic, and hormonal disturbances in women with and without polycystic ovary syndrome? Eur J Obstet Gynecol Reprod Biol. 2011;158:254–9.
12. Rustamov O, Krishnan M, Mathur R, Roberts S, Fitzgerald C. The effect of BMI on the ovarian reserve. British Fertility Society Annual Meeting; 2014.
13. Depmann M, Faddy MJ, van der Schouw YT, P. Peeters HM, Broer S, Kelsey TM, Nelson SM, Broekmans FJM. The relationship between variation in size of the primordial follicle pool and age at natural menopause. J Clin Endocrinol Metab. 2015;100(6):E845–51.
14. Durlinger AL, et al. Control of primordial follicle recruitment by anti-Mullerian hormone in the mouse ovary. Endocrinology. 1999;140(12):5789–96.
15. Durlinger AL, et al. Anti-Mullerian hormone attenuates the effects of FSH on follicle development in the mouse ovary. Endocrinology. 2001;142(11):4891–9.
16. Kelsey TW, et al. A validated model of serum anti-mullerian hormone from conception to menopause. PLoS One. 2011;6(7):e22024.
17. Templeton A, Morris JK, Parslow W. Factors that affect outcome of in-vitro fertilisation treatment. Lancet. 1996;348(9039):1402–6.
18. van Kooij RJ, et al. Age-dependent decrease in embryo implantation rate after in vitro fertilization. Fertil Steril. 1996;66(5):769–75.
19. Broekmans FJ, et al. A systematic review of tests predicting ovarian reserve and IVF outcome. Hum Reprod Update. 2006;12(6):685–718.
20. Abdalla H, Thum MY. Repeated testing of basal FSH levels has no predictive value for IVF outcome in women with elevated basal FSH. Hum Reprod. 2006;21(1):171–4.
21. Rustamov O, Pemberton P, Roberts S, Smith A, Yates A, Patchava S, Nardo L. The reproducibility of serum AMH in subfertile women: within and between patient variability. Fertil Steril. March 2011.
22. Broekmans Frank JM, de Ziegler D, Howles Colin M, Gougeon A, Trew G, Olivennes F. The antral follicle count: practical recommendations for better standardization. Fertil Steril. 2010;94:1044–51.

23. Jayaprakasan K, et al. A prospective, comparative analysis of anti-Mullerian hormone, inhibin-B, and three-dimensional ultrasound determinants of ovarian reserve in the prediction of poor response to controlled ovarian stimulation. Fertil Steril. 2010a;93(3):855–64.
24. Jayaprakasan K, et al. The cohort of antral follicles measuring 2–6 mm reflects the quantitative status of ovarian reserve as assessed by serum levels of anti-Mullerian hormone and response to controlled ovarian stimulation. Fertil Steril. 2010b;94:1775–81.
25. Haadsma ML, Bukman A, Groen H, Roeloffzen EM, Groenewoud ER, Heineman MJ, et al. The number of small antral follicles (2–6 mm) determines the outcome of endocrine ovarian reserve tests in a subfertile population. Hum Reprod. 2007;22:1925–31.
26. Rustamov O, Krishnan M, MacDougall J, Prentice A, Roberts S, Fitzgerald S, Mathur R. Antral follicle count: assessment of the discriminatory power of AFC by evaluation of its within-patient and between-patient variability. In: 9th Biennial Conference of UK Fertility Societies; 2015.
27. Rustamov O, Smith A, Roberts SA, et al. Anti-Mullerian hormone: poor assay reproducibility in a large cohort of subjects suggests sample instability. Hum Reprod. 2012;27:3085–91.
28. Yates AP, Rustamov O, Roberts SA, et al. Anti-Mullerian hormone-tailored stimulation protocols improve outcomes whilst reducing adverse effects and costs of IVF. Hum Reprod. 2011;26:2353–62.
29. Anderson RA. Pretreatmentserumanti-müllerianhormonepredicts long-term ovarian function and bone mass after chemotherapy for early breast cancer. J Clin Endocrinol Metab. 2011;96:1336–43.
30. Broer SL, Dólleman M, Opmeer BC, Fauser BC, Mol BW, Broekmans FJM. AMH and AFC as predictors of excessive response in controlled ovarian hyperstimulation: a meta-analysis. Hum Reprod Update. 2011a;17(1):46–54.
31. Broer SL, Eijkemans MJ, Scheffer GJ, et al. Anti-mullerianhormone predicts menopause: a long-term follow-up study in normoovulatory women. J Clin Endocrinol Metab. 2011b;96:2532–9.
32. Hudson PL, Dougas L, Donahoe PK, et al. An immunoassay to detect human müllerian inhibiting substance in males and females during normal development. J Clin Endocrinol Metab. 1990;70:16–22.
33. Qin Y, Jiao X, Simpson JL, Chen ZJ. Genetics of primary ovarian insufficiency: new developments and opportunities. Hum Reprod Update. 2015;21(6):787–808.
34. American College of Obstetricians and Gynecologists Committee on Genetics. ACOG committee opinion No. 469: carrier screening for fragile X syndrome. Obstet Gynecol. 2010;116(4):1008–10.
35. Strom CM, Crossley B, Redman JB, Buller A, Quan F, Peng M, McGinnis M, Fenwick RG Jr, Sun W. Molecular testing for Fragile X Syndrome: lessons learned from 119,232 tests performed in a clinical laboratory. Genet Med. 2007;9(1):46–51.
36. Edwards JG, Feldman G, Goldberg J, Gregg AR, Norton ME, Rose NC, Schneider A, Stoll K, Wapner R, Watson MS. Expanded carrier screening in reproductive medicine-points to consider: a joint statement of the American College of Medical Genetics and Genomics, American College of Obstetricians and Gynecologists, National Society of Genetic Counselors, Perinatal Quality Foundation, and Society for Maternal-Fetal Medicine. Obstet Gynecol. 2015;125(3):653–62.
37. Henneman L, Borry P, Chokoshvili D, Cornel MC, van El CG, Forzano F, Hall A, Howard HC, Janssens S, Kayserili H, Lakeman P, Lucassen A, Metcalfe SA, Vidmar L, de Wert G, Dondorp WJ, Peterlin B. Responsible implementation of expanded carrier screening. Eur J Hum Genet. 2016;24(6):e1–12.

Chapter 5
Alternative Options for Preventive Oocyte Cryopreservation

Marja Visser

Introduction

Since contraception became more accessible in the 1970s of the last century, women came in the position to postpone her first pregnancy [1]. Next to the accessibility to effective contraception, education of women, gender equity and partnership changes, but also economic uncertainty and the absence of supportive family policies delayed motherhood [2–4]. About 30 years ago women gave birth to their first child at the age of 24.1; nowadays this is at the age of 29.4 [5]. Women postpone their desire for a child due to lack of a partner or due to a career despite their wish, or they prioritize an independent life [4, 6]. To circumvent age-related fertility decline, women can opt for banking their oocytes. This gives them the possibility of potential shared parenthood in future, regardless the perceived health risks and psychosocial implications [7]. Women who bank their oocytes to have more time to find the right partner decide a few years after the vitrification to choose for single motherhood and donor sperm treatment (about 14%) [8]. When single women do not opt for banking their oocytes and/or they do not find a partner to start a family, women consider starting their own family without a partner. Most single women wish to have a nuclear family in future, but an increasingly amount of women seek for an unconventional family formation to become a mother, such as sperm donation, adoption or fostering [9]. Since a few decades there has been a significant rise of single women opting for donor sperm treatment [10–12].

M. Visser
Academic Medical Center, University of Amsterdam,
Q4-123, Meibergdreef 9, Amsterdam, 1105 AZ, The Netherlands
e-mail: M.Visser@amc.uva.nl

© Springer International Publishing Switzerland 2018

D. Stoop (ed.), *Preventing Age Related Fertility Loss*,
DOI 10.1007/978-3-319-14857-1_5

Becoming a Mom with the Help of Donor Sperm

Becoming a mom can be such a strong desire that a lot of single women in their 30s do not want to wait any longer to find a partner for building their own family. They no longer want to postpone their wish to get pregnant and choose to be a single mom with the help of a sperm donor. They often believe that finding a partner will always be possible at an older age, but for getting pregnant this might be too late.

Many women who choose this option register at a fertility clinic. They opt for a sperm donor of a sperm bank and the help of medical professionals and some psychosocial guidance in this process [13]. Other women who feel that it is important to know the donor/(donor)-father of their child, try to find a donor themselves and start with self-inseminations at home. Some of them ask a good friend being the (donor)-father, but others prefer someone from outside their inner circle such as a friend of someone with whom they are familiar. There are also women who seek a (donor)-father for co-parenting, as they find it important that their future child will have a father. These women choose for a homosexual man being the (donor)-father or a homosexual couple, as these men also may have a wish for building a family. Actually, these women and men seek a father or a mother for their future child.

Until 1985 sperm donors were anonymous and couples were advised to keep the sperm donation a secret to their child [14, 15]. Identifiable sperm donation came more into focus in addition to anonymous donation in those years. Several countries such as Sweden, the Netherlands, the United Kingdom, Switzerland, Germany, New Zealand and Australia have prohibited anonymity of sperm donors. These countries have developed specific laws to allow donor-conceived offspring to learn about the identity of their donors from adolescence. In Spain, Czech Republic and France sperm donors are obliged to be anonymous and in some countries such as Belgium and Denmark sperm donors both can be anonymous or identifiable. Women also have the possibility to buy donor sperm from a foreign sperm bank and either inseminates themselves or seek a fertility clinic or medical doctor to assist them with the inseminations.

The societal debate on the options of anonymity or identifiability had been polarised between the "right to privacy" of the parent and the "right to know" of the donor-conceived child. At the same time the debate on secrecy and disclosure to donor-children came more into focus. Opinions, policies and outcomes of research contributed to this debate. Gradually became clearer that when parents share donor conception with their child, they experience fewer emotional problems and have a more open communication with each other and their child [15–18]. Donor-children who have been studied find it important that their parents are honest about donor conception and wish to be informed about their genetic origins and about the identity of the donor [18–22].

The Sperm Donor

When women are dependent on sperm from a donor of a sperm bank, they have clear wishes with respect to the donor [24]. Most women prefer to have a say in the selection of the sperm donor. At least they want to know his motivation, as knowing his motivation gives women a closer idea of his personality. They also prefer a donor with a social personality, as they value this as important for the identity of their future child. Another feature that women appreciate is that the donor is intelligent and that he has followed a higher education. Women also prefer that his appearance is similar to theirs, as they feel when a child is close to the mother, this is less difficult for the child. There are also women who do not wish to have a say in this selection for a donor, as this would give them a kind of responsibility they do not like.

Women who choose for an identifiable sperm donor assume that once their child wants to meet the donor. They want to enable this with their choice and also feel that they should facilitate the contact of the child with him at that time. A main concern regarding future contact with the donor is that the expectations of their child and the sperm donor will not be the same, and their child could be disappointed by that. Women also are thinking about issues as what could happen when that their child would fall in love with his half sibling and when the donor already has passed away when their child would like to meet the donor. They put effort in finding the right fertility clinic and think about choosing for an identifiable donor, for an anonymous donor or for a donor they can know themselves.

Psychosocial Implications and Counselling

One of the reasons for women to choose for an anonymous sperm donor is that it will be easier for their future child not to face the choice whether to meet the donor or not from the age of 16 or 18 or to be disappointed about the donor. They wish to protect their child from harm. There are also women who choose for an identifiable donor, as they find it important that their future child has the possibility to have contact with the donor. These women feel that a child has the right to know the donor, and that this will be important for his/her identity (Dusseldorp et al., unpublished data). These women also choose for sharing donor conception from an early age as they do not want to have a secret for their child. It is suggested that single women do not have the opportunity to keep donor conception a secret for their child. But when they feel ashamed towards people around them and/or guilty towards their child for withholding them a father, women may hesitate to share donor conception with their child and postpone disclosure [23].

Women appreciate the availability of specialist counselling to talk about the implications for themselves and for their child. Psychosocial counselling before donor sperm treatment is often part of the treatment procedure in fertility clinics. It offers women the opportunity to discuss their decision whether or not to start with donor sperm treatment and/or to discuss the implications of becoming a single mom by using donor sperm treatment. During the intake procedure they also can be informed about practice experiences and research outcomes. This can be information about the influence on the wellbeing of children growing up without a father, about sharing with children about their genetic origins and how to talk about the donor. Women appreciate the opportunity of having contact with a specialist counsellor if they need counselling in the future [23].

Women often seek contact with other single women who want to get children alone, or feel that they would appreciate such contact in future. In some countries as the United Kingdom, Australia, Germany and the Netherlands women can follow workshops with other single women to give support in the decision making process becoming a single mom and/or preparing them for single motherhood with the help of a sperm donor [24].

Preparing for Single Motherhood

Many single women attending to sperm donation are high-educated, older than women with a male partner when they want to get pregnant and they have a good financial positions and good social networks [17, 25]. These women have a wish to get children, but are ambivalent to choose for single motherhood as most of them prefer building a family with a partner they love [9]. They feel that single motherhood is not 'natural' and it is 'Plan-B' to get pregnant either with the help of a donor they know themselves, or with the help of an unknown donor of a sperm bank. Therefore, women take time to prepare for single motherhood. They think it over from at least 1 year to a very long time before they make the decision (Dusseldorp et al., unpublished data). They often discuss their thoughts and feelings extensively with family and friends and sometimes they discuss single motherhood with a psychologist or with their physician. Important factors in preparing for single motherhood are financial security, emotional stability and having a supportive social network [17, 25].

One of the most important concerns of many single women is the absence of a father for their future child. They feel this as a failure and women fear that not knowing who the father is would influence the identity of their future child [24]. Many women think about a male role model for their child to fill the gap of the missing father. Another concern is that not having a partner may lead to feelings of loneliness. They realize that they are the only ones who will be responsible for the child and that they will not be able to discuss doubts and sharing special moments of their child with a father.

In contrast with those concerns, women also expect benefits of being a single mom, as not having to take a partners' opinion into account during the sperm donation process or during raising their future child. Another benefit is that they felt that a child would not experience any divorce of the parents, as in their opinion a divorce or separation would be more detrimental for a child than having a single mother from birth on [24].

Single Motherhood and the Wellbeing of Children

High education and an older age of single mothers are suggested to be protective factors for stability. Studies on parental conflict in father-absent families—i.e. the father has been present in the past-reveal that parent-child conflicts in father-absent families can be a strong influential factor on emotional distress of children conceived after donor sperm treatment [25]. Although, negative outcomes in those studies cannot necessarily be generalized to single-mother families formed after donor sperm treatment [17, 26, 27]. A longitudinal study on children of single women confirms the theory that donor-children of single women are not compromised comparing to their peers of from father-mother families [28–30]. In those studies, no negative consequences for the parent-child relationship or psychological adjustment of children of single mothers were found.

Single women have high expectations regarding their own motherhood and their ability to provide a solid basis for a child, but they also have fear for possible consequences. For both heterosexual and lesbian couples who use donor sperm to build a family, but also for single women it is of value to have access to trustful information, to contact with (intended) single mothers to share experiences and learn from each other and to specialist professional counselling and guidance to gain support as much as possible.

Alternative Options for Women to Get a Family without Own Gametes

When women do not opt for banking their oocytes and/or donor sperm treatment there are several other options to start a family.

Co-parenting without having a partner-relationship. As well as women and men, hetero- and homosexual seek to have a family and getting children together.

Adoption and fostering are possibilities open for single women. Since 2011 in the Netherlands 74 children were adopted by single women, ranging from 7 children until 18 children per year. They adopted children from several continents, from China, the USA, Africa and European countries. In the Netherlands the selection rules are stricter than for couples and more women need psychosocial guidance for themselves or for their child [31].

Going without children is an option for women who do not want to have children without a partner-relationship and for women who do not have a wish to get children at all.

Keynotes

1. There is an increasing rise of single women opting for donor sperm treatment the last decade.
2. Single women who choose for donor sperm treatment made a step forward in becoming a single mom compared to single women who are banking their oocytes.
3. One of the greatest concerns: the negative consequences for a child to grow up without a father.
4. Specialist psychosocial guidance and trustful network organizations for fellow support should be available and further developed.
5. Living without children can also be a thoughtful choice for single women.

References

1. Beets G, Dourleijn E, Liefbroer A, Henkens K. De timing van het eerste kind in Nederland en Europa. NIDI 2001, rapport 59, Den Haag.
2. Mills M, Rindfuss RR, McDonald P, te Velde E, Reproduction ESHRE, Force ST. Why do people postpone parenthood? Reasons and social policy incentives. Hum Reprod Update. 2011;17(6):848–60.
3. Johnson JA, Tough S. Society of obstetricians and gynaecologists of Canada. Delayed childbearing. J Obstet Gynaecol Can. 2012;34:80–93.
4. Schmidt L, Sobotka T, Bentzen JG, Andersen AN. Demographic and medical consequences of the postponement of parenthood. Hum Reprod Update. 2012;18:29–43.
5. Centraal Bureau voor de Statistiek (CBS). 2017. https://www.cbs.nl/nl-nl/faq/specifiek/worden-vrouwen-steeds-ouder-moeder. Accessed 7 Feb 2017.
6. Schytt E, Nilsen AB, Bernhardt E. Still childless at the age of 28 to 40 years: a cross-sectional study of Swedish women's and men's reproductive intentions. Sex Reprod Healthc. 2014;5(1):23–9.
7. Groot de M, Dancet E, Repping S, Goddijn M, Stoop D, van der Veen F, Gerrits T. Perceptions of oocyte banking from women intending to circumvent age-related fertility decline. Acta Obstet Gynecol Scand. 2016;95(12):1396–401.
8. Balkenende E, Dahhan S, Goddijn M, Repping S, van der Veen F. Reproductive outcome after oocyte banking for fertility preservation.
9. Peterson KB, Sylvest R, Andersen AN, Pinborg A, Hvidman HW, Schmidt L. Attitudes towards family formation in cohabiting and single childless women in their mid- to late thirties. Hum Fertil. 2016;19(1):48–55.
10. Viloria T, Garrido N, Minaya F, Remohi J, Munoz M, Meseguer M. Report of results obtained in 2,934 women using donor sperm: donor insemination versus in vitro fertilization according to indication. Fertil Steril. 2011;96(5):1134–7.
11. Fiske Emily WG. Utilisation of ART in single women and lesbian couples since the 2010 change in victorian legislation. Aust N Z J Obstet Gynaecol. 2014;54:497–9.
12. Kop PA, van Wely M, Mol BW, de Melker AA, Janssens PM, Arends B, Curfs MH, Kortman M, Nap A, Rijnders E, Roovers JP, Ruis H, Simons AH, Repping S, van der Veen F, Mochtar MH. Intrauterine insemination or intracervical insemination with cryopreserved donor sperm in the natural cycle: a cohort study. Hum Reprod. 2015;30(3):603–7.
13. ESHRE Taskforce on Ethics and Law. III. Gamete and embryo donation. Hum Reprod. 2002;17(5):1407–8.
14. Lalos A, Gottlieb C, Lalos O. Legislated right for donor-insemination children to know their genetic origin: a study of parental thinking. Hum Reprod. 2007;22(6):1759–68.
15. Rumball A, Adair V. Telling the story: parents' scripts for donor offspring. Hum Reprod. 1999;14(5):1392–9.
16. van den Akker O. A review of family donor constructs: current research and future directions. Hum Reprod Update. 2006;12(2):91–101. Review
17. Jadva V, Badger S, Morrissette M, Golombok S. 'Mom by choice, single by life's circumstance...' Findings from a large scale survey of the experiences of single mothers by choice. Hum Fertil (Camb). 2009;12(4):175–84.
18. Scheib JE, Riordan M, Rubin S. Adolescents with open-identity sperm donors: reports from 12-17 year olds. Hum Reprod. 2005;20(1):239–52.
19. Turner AJ, Coyle A. What does it mean to be a donor offspring? The identity experiences of adults conceived by donor insemination and the implications for counselling and therapy. Hum Reprod. 2000;15(9):2041–51.
20. Berger R, Paul M. Family secrets and family functioning: the case of donor assistance. Fam Process. 2008;47:553–66.
21. Beeson DR, Jennings PK, Kramer W. Offspring searching for their sperm donors: how family type shapes the process. Hum Reprod. 2011;26:2415–24.

22. Blyth E, Crawshaw M, Frith L, Jones C. Donor-conceived people's views and experiences of their genetic origins: a critical analysis of the research evidence. J Law Med. 2012;19(4):769–89. Review
23. Visser M, Gerrits T, Kop F, der v, Veen F, Mochtar M. Exploring parents' feelings on psychosocial counseling in donor sperm treatment. J Psychosom Obstet Gynaecol. 2016;24:1–8.
24. Dusseldorp F, Visser M and Mochtar M. Unpublished data; 2015.
25. Yap MBH, Jorm AF. Parental factors associated with childhood anxiety, depression, and internalizing problems: a systematic review and meta-analysis. J Affect Disord. 2015;1(175):424–40.
26. Ethics Committee of the American Society for Reproductive Medicine. Informing offspring of their conception by gamete or embryo donation: a committee opinion. Fertil Steril. 2013;100:45–9.
27. Practice committe of the American Society for Reproductive Medicine and Practice Committee of the Society for Assisted Reproductive Technology. Recommendations for gamete and embryo donation; A committee opinion. Fertil Steril. 2013;99(1):47–62.
28. Maccallum F, Golombok S. Children raised in fatherless families from infancy: a follow-up of children of lesbian and single heterosexual mothers at early adolescence. J Child Psychol Pscyhiatry. 2004;45(8):1407–19.
29. Murray C, Golombok S. Solo mothers and their donor insemination infants: follow-up at age 2 years. Hum Reprod. 2005;20(6):1655–60.
30. Golombok S, Tasker FMF. Children raised in fatherless families from infancy: family relationships and the socioemotional development of children of lesbian and single heterosexual mothers. J Child Psychol Psychiatry. 1997;38(7):783–91.
31. Stichting Adoptie Voorzieningen. 2016. http://www.adoptie.nl/

Chapter 6
The Profile of a Pioneer Cohort of Women Opting for Oocyte Cryopreservation for Non-medical Reasons

Julie Nekkebroeck

Introduction

Since 2009 the Centre for Reproductive Medicine of the UZ Brussel offers the possibility to women in anticipation of gamete exhaustion (AGE) [1] to cryopreserve their oocytes. The onset took place in an era of societal and political debate (e.g. The Netherlands) and warnings by the main professional organizations in the area of reproductive medicine [2, 3] especially about the non-medical use of oocyte cryopreservation. For instance, the American Society of Reproductive Medicine [2] stated that oocyte cryopreservation is an "experimental procedure" that should not be offered or marketed as a means to defer reproductive aging. The British Fertility Society (BFS) agrees that oocyte cryopreservation should not be portrayed as a means to counteract age related fertility decline [3].

What was initially offered to women faced with illness or medical treatment resulting in infertility is nowadays a treatment that is (luckily) more often used for non-medical indications leading many ethicists in the area of reproduction to examine the benefits and pitfalls of this application. Objections formulated against AGE-banking are that; the whole process of reproduction becomes medicalized and perhaps even commercialized undermining rather than expanding women's reproductive autonomy [4]. Moreover, healthy women have to undergo a stress-inducing high technological fertility treatment without having an actual fertility problem and little is known about the welfare of the children born after the use of cryopreserved oocytes. One also assumes that women will deliberately postpone motherhood until the time of their choosing, that women will give priority to their careers and that oocyte cryopreservation will offer a false sense of security that one is optimizing her chances of motherhood [4].

J. Nekkebroeck
Department of Developmental and Lifespan Psychology, Centre for Reproductive Medicine, UZ Brussel, Vrije Universiteit Brussel, Laarbeeklaan 101, Brussel 1090, Belgium
e-mail: Julie.nekkebroeck@uzbrussel.be

© Springer International Publishing Switzerland 2018
D. Stoop (ed.), *Preventing Age Related Fertility Loss*,
DOI 10.1007/978-3-319-14857-1_6

In contrast, those in favour of AGE-banking for non-medical reasons stress the possible benefits for women and their right to ascertain reproductive autonomy after comprehensive counselling. More precisely, personal reproductive decisions should be free from interference unless they will cause serious harm to others. Another argument in favour of AGE-banking for non-medical reasons is that it alleviates gender inequality by allowing women to extend their reproductive years just as men are able to do already for many decades. As such, women should also gain access to this technology that will offer them this possibility to preserve their fertility [5]. Furthermore, this practice might be beneficial to the future child since it will be conceived when women feel ready, have a stable relationship and are financially secure but most importantly, the child will have a biological bond with his mother. Another advantage of oocyte cryopreservation instead of embryo cryopreservation is that it empowers women because it makes them less dependent of their partner and it allows her to have a child with a partner of her choosing [5].

Regardless of the societal and political debate oocyte cryopreservation seems only to elicit interest in a small niche of the female population. In a large survey ($n > 1000$), [6] only 3% of the women stated they were going to freeze oocytes. There was another 28.5% who was interested and considered oocyte freezing. This added up to 31.5% 'potential freezers'. In another study [7] only 4% of the women who inquire by phone at the Extend Fertility centre, Boston, USA about the fertility preservation treatment go on to use the technique. Ter Keurst et al. [8] who investigated the intentions of childless women aged between 28 and 35 years to use fertility preservation stated that 85% had thought about fertility preservation but only 4.6% had actually made a decision about it. Authors conclude that in general women have a low intention to use fertility preservation despite being childless, having a desire for a (genetically related) child, being in the age range when fertility starts to decline and having reasonable fertility knowledge. They relate these low intentions to three main issues; 'lack of perceived susceptibility to infertility' and 'defining overly optimistic parenthood goals' by giving themselves around 3 years to have two children (from 34.4 to 37.6 years). 'Failure to consider the use of fertility preservation' is the third issue. To explain this third factor they point to the work of Rogers [9] of 1962 about the diffusion of innovations. According to him the first stage of diffusion happens when individuals know about the technology but have not been inspired to get more precise information. So knowing that fertility preservation exists women tend not to find out more about it (e.g. take contact with a fertility centre). Another way to define this failure is the fact that women might rely on ART with fresh oocytes to overcome fertility problems. However, older women felt more susceptible to infertility and had higher intentions to use fertility preservation.

Besides the fact that only a small niche of the female population seems to be interested it is also striking that when women actually candidate to become an AGE banker they do this at a suboptimal age—in their late 30s—when oocyte reserve and quality strongly diminished and pregnancy rates drop significantly [10]. According to Ter Keurst et al. [8], the knowledge of the candidate AGE-banker on fertility issues is reasonable but may lack precision about fertility decline and the success of fertility preservation. Women might only feel susceptible to infertility at this age while not realising that at that time fertility preservation rates are not optimal which is reflected in the lack of a feasible parenthood plan. The main preventive measure these authors propose is for health care professionals and policy makers to increase fertility awareness and support women in creating a realistic plan to achieve parenthood goals via educational campaigns or family planning consultations. Mertes and Pennings [10] discern three different steps to make the current practice of oocyte cryopreservation more clinically and ethically sound: creating public awareness; offering individualized, age-specific information and counselling; and offering predictive tests such as anti-Müllerian hormone measurements and antral follicle count. The main objective of these measures is to convince those women who are most likely to benefit from banking in AGE to present themselves before age 35 and to discourage fertility clinics from specifically targeting women who have already surpassed the age at which good results can be expected all this not to install false hope in reproductively older women.

Studies examining the actual AGE-banker and her motivation(s) to opt for this procedure could challenge the speculations and assumptions made about this specific population but are still scarce anno 2017. A study [11] reported on a small number of women (n = 20) wanting to cryopreserve their oocytes for non-medical reasons. These women were on average 38.6 years old and often they were single and had a high educational level. Wanting to take advantage of all possible reproductive opportunities feeling pressured by their biological clock and wanting an 'insurance policy' against future age-related infertility were the main reasons for opting for oocyte cryopreservation. The pivotal events to apply for the treatment were the recent awareness of the existence of the technique; their advanced reproductive age and not wanting to single parent a child. Another study [12] also reported on a small group of women (n = 23) who froze their oocytes. On average they were 36.7 years old, mostly university educated, 87% was single and 88% was prepared to donate there eggs for research or to women in need of donor eggs in case they would not use there eggs. Their motivation to cryopreserve oocytes was very similar to the motivations reported in the Gold-study but 1/5 also saw it as a preventive measure against age related fertility decline or other medical issues that would make them infertile (e.g. cancer treatment).

Hodes-Wertz [13] described the largest cohort of women post oocyte cryopreservation. One hundred and eighty three patients out of 478 (38%) participated in a survey follow-study. At the time of oocyte cryopreservation more than 80% was aged 35 years or older. Women were aware of the age related infertility and wished they had undergone the procedure at an earlier age. Unawareness of the technology and/or readily availability followed by not being ready and not being concerned about their reproductive future or unable to afford it were the reasons they gave for not acting sooner. They also felled that the popular media falsely portrayed the upper age limit for natural conception and 19% of the respondents added that workplace inflexibility contributed to their reproductive dilemma. However, "having no partner at the time to conceive with" was the main reason to pursue oocyte cryopreservation.

Counselling AGE-Bankers

In order to get acquainted with the candidates for AGE-banking (for non-medical reasons) these women were systematically counselled in accordance with the recommendations by the main professional bodies (ASRM and BFS and later ESHRE [14]). Counselling was performed by a gynaecologist and a psychologist in a non-directive manner with respect for reproductive autonomy making sure that realistic expectations are being created and that well-informed decisions can be made about oocyte cryopreservation an whether to proceed with the treatment or not.

All candidates underwent a semi-structured interview performed by a psychologist in which the following topics were addressed: socio-demographics, mental health, relationships and child desire, discovery of the possibility to cryopreserve oocytes, initial motives to opt for this treatment and/or alternatives, openness about this project towards family, friends and the received support, the possible disadvantages, risks and limitations of the treatment and the use of the cryopreserved oocytes.

A minor medical assessment was performed by a gynaecologist and blood samples were taken in order to evaluate hormone levels (FSH and AMH) and an antral follicle count was performed.

Between July 2009 and December 2012, 243 women contacted the Centre for Reproductive Medicine with the intention to freeze their oocytes. Not all of them had already made the decision to actually freeze oocytes and for many of them it was unsure whether it would medically/physically feasible and responsible to perform this treatment because of their advanced reproductive age. About half of the women (n = 124 or 51%) went through with the treatment although for four candidates (1.6%) oocyte pick-up had to be cancelled because of a low response.

One hundred and nineteen candidates (49%) did not start treatment; 21 candidates were refused for treatment usually because they were over 40 years old, 14 candidates hormones levels were unfavourable to start treatment, 20 candidates stated at the intake that they were still undecided whether they would start the treatment, for 22 candidates it remained unclear why they did not take upon treatment and 33 (13.6%) candidates did not go through with the treatment for 'other reasons' (e.g. 4 became pregnant spontaneously, 9 found a partner, 9 made a switch to another treatment, 6 found it too expensive, 5 mentioned other reasons not to perform treatment). On average these patients underwent 1.83 (±1.06) oocyte pick-ups and have 15.96 (±9.8) oocytes in the freezer.

Counselling these women also allowed us to document on the profile of this population. Data are presented from women who did not only apply for treatment but who also actually went through with the treatment (n = 124).

Socio-Demographics

Women were of an advanced reproductive age, on average 36.74 (±2.59) years old, highly educated (70.2% university degree, 28.2% degree) full time employed (79.8%) and mostly Dutch speaking (73.4%) according to their Dutch (57.3%) or Belgian (18.5%) nationality.

Mental Health and Relationships

Almost all women (97.6%) had had relationships in the past and at the time of the intake the majority (82.3%) was single. About 38.1% experienced a relationship break-up the past year and 16.1% women had one or more abortions in the past while none of the women already had a child. 20.2% did follow some form of therapy (psychotherapy or psychotropic medication or a combination) usually in the context of relational suffering e.g. to deal with a (recent) break-up, to reflect on why they had such a hard time finding the right partner.

Desire for a Child Versus Desire for a Partner

At present, 19.5% of the women did not feel a very outspoken desire for a child, 39.9% felt this desire only since a few years and 40.7% stated they always had pictured themselves as future mothers. So, not surprisingly more than one third (42.7%) of the women felt at this moment in time a stronger desire for a partner than that they felt the need to fulfil their desire for a child (5.6%). However, for one-third (34.7%) both desires were strongly connected. The main explanatory factor as to why they did not have children yet was the fact they did not find the right partner yet to have children with (62.9%). Only 4% stated they gave full priority to their career, 5.6% was undecided about whether they wanted to have children or not, in other cases the (ex-) partner did not have a desire for a child (anymore) or a combination of the above factors were mentioned as the reason why they did not have children yet.

Discovery of the Possibility and Motives to Cryopreserve Oocytes

One third of the women (36.6%) had discovered the possibility to freeze oocytes because the topic appeared in the media or by searching on the internet (11.4%). Age bankers started to network as well, through the internet but also in the waiting room of the fertility clinic and many of the women who candidate today for age banking know somebody who also had this treatment or is interested in having it. For 22% the possibility to cryopreserve oocytes was pointed out to them by friends, colleagues or relatives.

The main reasons to candidate for this treatment were: assurance against future age-related infertility (55.6%), buying more time to find that right partner (37.9%) and taking the pressure of the search for a suitable partner (29%). Another 28.2% of the women also saw the benefits of this treatment in the light of new or future relationships. By cryopreserving their oocytes they stated they could give their relationships more time to blossom before bringing up the subject of child-desire, hereby avoiding putting pressure on their partner and/or relationship. A less important reason to perform oocyte cryopreservation was the idea of having tried everything by taking advantage of all possible (reproductive) opportunities to preserve their fertility (26.6%).

Alternatives

Before the possibility of oocyte cryopreservation was discovered; adoption or staying childless were considered as alternatives by respectively 16.9% and 10.5% of the women. Becoming a single mother with the use of either anonymous or known donor sperm was a more popular alternative, considered by approximately one third (33.1%) of the women but rather as a last resort at a very advanced reproductive age. Only 1.6% would consider conception after a one-night stand and 4.8% stated they have no alternatives in mind if they could not freeze their oocytes. However, clearly for most women (84.7%) actively keep on searching for 'mister right' was the only valuable option in order to avoid single parenthood and the need for donor eggs at an older reproductive age. 65.3% also actively engaged in the search for a partner by visiting dating sites, consulting dating agencies and by addressing their social network (19.2%). 17.7% already has a relationship at the moment of intake (early or established >6 months) while 16.9% is not actively engaging in finding a suitable partner.

Attitudes and Concerns

None of the women who cryopreserved oocytes formulated any moral, religious or ethical objections about oocyte cryopreservation for non-medical reasons and the majority stated they had no problem with the fact they had to undergo a fertility treatment while being considered healthy and/or fertile and they accepted that at present little information is available on the well-being of the children born after oocyte cryopreservation.

Disadvantages of the Oocyte Cryopreservation

The use of hormones (44.4%) and the financial costs (21%) were considered as the main disadvantages of the treatment. Less mentioned disadvantages were: the concern that the treatment will be a physical or a psychological burden (8.1%), the fact that one has to undergo a fertility treatment (4%), the fact that the treatment does not offer any guarantees on childbearing (7.3%), the practical arrangements that need to be made (16.9%) and some personal fears that had to be overcome before engaging in this treatment (e.g. fear of stigmatization, gynaecological examination, fear that their oocytes would be switched with those of other patients).

Openness and Support from the Social Network

The overall majority of the women (98.4%) had shared their intentions to cryopreserve oocytes with at least one person in their entourage and none of them felt discouraged to undergo this treatment. Reactions were positive (82%) or mixed (18%) as some people showed some concern about the fact that their daughter/relative/friend was about to undergo a treatment. However, 22.6% did not tell their parents about their plans to cryopreserve their oocytes and in 13.7% of the cases the father was not informed. Because they did not want to worry them, they were undecided at intake about continuing this treatment or they wanted first to make sure they got the permission of the centre to freeze oocytes. In contrast, two patients stated they were embarrassed to tell their parents because they believed their parents would prefer them to have children the traditional way by first finding a suitable partner, getting married and have children the natural way. By cryopreserving their oocytes it felt as if they were failing in the eyes of their parents. About 8.1% stated they would have no support during treatment -amongst which a few women who actually preferred 'to do this on their own' (n = 6). All of the others stated they would get support from their entourage during treatment. With this support they meant they would find someone that would accompany them to the clinic (73.4%) the day of oocyte retrieval and 17.7%, will not only be accompanied to the clinic but will also get financial support. In case women have a partner, 77.2% tells the partner about the plans to undergo a treatment. In our sample 22 women had an ongoing relationship and 17 partners knew about the plans of their partner.

Treatment Aspects

76.6% stated they could afford different treatment cycles, which cost about 2500 euro per cycle including medication, oocyte pick-up and 10 years of oocyte cryopreservation.

However, the other 23.4% stated it would not be possible to pay for a second treatment cycle. On average they wanted to repeat the treatment 1.83 times (±1.06) and the average age women thought of using their oocytes was 42.73 years with a SD of 2.51 years.

However, the actual decision to repeat the treatment would depend on how the first treatment was experienced and on the number of oocytes cryopreserved after the first treatment cycle.

Use of the Cryopreserved Oocytes

If they would find a suitable partner most of them would want to try to become pregnant spontaneously, than perform IVF with fresh collected material and in last instance, perform IVF with their cryopreserved oocytes (86.3%). 3.2% would because of their age at present immediately use the vitrified oocytes and 8.9% would first ask doctor's advice before deciding what to do. If they would no longer need their oocytes 22% was unsure about their destination at the time of intake or 4.9% was sure that they would certainly not let them get destroyed, 33.3% would donate them for scientific research, 15.4% would let them get destroyed and 19.6% stated they would donate them anonymously or known to a woman with fertility problems.

The Profile of the Pioneer Cohort of Women Opting for Oocyte Cryopreservation

When we summarize the results obtained from this group of women we may state that women who bank oocytes in anticipation of gamete exhaustion (AGE) are highly educated single women of an older reproductive age, struggling with relationships but having a strong desire for a partner that momentarily beats their desire for a child. They want to fond a family with this suitable partner and raise a child in the presence of a father. Although most women are highly educated and have a career only a very small percentage attributes the fact that they do not have children yet to the deliberate postponement of the realization of their desire for a child in function of a career. A recent break-up, advanced reproductive age, awareness of the possibility were the pivotal events to candidate for treatment. Well aware of the importance not to solely relay on this possibility to attain their reproductive goal, the majority of the women actively or more passively engaged in finding a suitable partner. By cryopreserving their oocytes they wanted to buy more time to find that partner, relieve the pressure of the search for a partner and take an insurance against future age-related infertility. In general women seemed to be well aware of the risks and limitations of the treatment but were not stressed out about them or did not feel discouraged. Most of the time able to afford different treatment cycles the financial cost was one of the main disadvantages of the treatment besides the need to use hormones. These financial and physical efforts they have to make might contribute to the fact that cryopreserved oocytes are considered as precious goods that will only be used in last instance, after having tried to become pregnant spontaneously and/or having performed a fresh IVF cycle. Moreover, these vitrified oocytes are also considered to be very personal goods. In case they do not need them, the majority would prefer to donate them for scientific research or let them get destroyed rather than to donate them anonymously (or known) to women in need of donor eggs.

Discussion

The assessed cohort of women represents a very homogenous group possibly related to the descriptive nature of the study and to the pioneer population involved. The population of women opting the cryopreserve oocytes may become more diverse as the indication for oocyte cryopreservation would become more common. In the general population of women of a reproductive age, women were found to be concerned about financial costs, health risks for themselves and a future child, the impact of hormones and success rates linked to oocyte cryopreservation making them more reluctant towards the possibility [15]. The actual age-banker in our cohort seems to be much less worried about those aspects and wants to grasp the opportunity to prevail (what is left of) her fertility. Possibly, only a very specific niche of the female population might benefit from this treatment and is interested in having it.

It is clear that the profile of these women needs to be considered preliminary and further follow-up is needed. This pioneer cohort of women seems to be functioning well on a cognitive level according to their educational levels and engagement in employment. Although all these women are highly educated and have a career, it is confirmed that women attribute their childlessness to 'not having met a suitable partner' rather than to 'prioritisation of career achievements'. At the relational/emotional level more instability and suffering is noticed. Starting a relationship is not a problem for this cohort, it is the long-term establishment that seems not to be evident; partners do not live up to their expectations, often it is stated that the partners in the past were "not ideal" to have a child with, regularly a discrepancy is mentioned in the desire for a child between them and the past or current partner and also a reproach of a lack of engagement of the (ex-) partner is frequently reported. Women often seek psychotherapy in order to address these relational issues.

The profile of the women in our cohort seems to be very similar to those described by other authors [11–13]. Unfortunately, the women in our cohort also cryopreserved oocytes at a suboptimal reproductive age (mean 36.95 years). Concurrently, to offering women the possibility to cryopreserve oocytes, efforts to promote change in social and political structures in order to eliminate discriminatory features of society should be made. Mertes and Pennings [10] promote; creating public awareness; having children at a younger reproductive age and offering individualized, age-specific information and counselling and predictive tests (anti-Müllerian hormone measurements or antral follicle count) in order to help women to create realistic expectations and to make well-informed decisions. As a result from counselling, women may have a realistic view on the treatment aspects (pitfalls and limitation) however, they may (still) have unrealistic expectations about partners and relationships. Wanting to cryopreserve oocytes in their late 30s, still hoping for prince charming to come along and only willing to accomplish the desire for a child with this "perfect" partner may not be very realistic. What are the chances of finding this partner in the coming 5 years when they have not met him over the past 20 years? For some women age banking at an older reproductive age also means they will be flirting with the legal age limit in Belgium for embryo transfer, which is set at age 47. The question remains how many women will be able to benefit from age banking and use it for what they intend to use it, namely, buying time to find the right partner and to fond a family. On the other hand, a significant amount of women—usually the reproductively speaking, older women—in our cohort (aged 38, 39) also consider the possibility of becoming a single parent, hereby showing a more realistic perspective on their reproductive options.

Continued follow-up of this cohort is necessary in order to have a better view on the trajectory of these women and to refine counselling at intake. More research exploring the personality features of these women is needed for a better understanding of this population. Moreover, results need to be analysed in relation to the societal, financial, educational demands and changes in Western society, making it hard for women to achieve important life goals (establish a career, finding a partner, having children) within a short timeframe, between the age of 30 and 40 when fertility has already declined.

Key Points Women who cryopreserve oocytes:

1. Are often single and do not have children (yet) because they did not meet the right partner to have children with not because they prioritise their career achievements
2. Have the desire to start a family rather than to single parent a child
3. Function well professionally and are financially independent but experience more relational suffering
4. Should be counselled prior to treatment preferably by a psychologist in a non-directive manner with respect for reproductive autonomy and a gynaecologist who provides individualized, age-specific information, in order to make sure that realistic expectations are being created and that well-informed decisions can be made by the candidate about oocyte cryopreservation and whether to proceed with the treatment or not
5. Do this at an advanced reproductive age when fertility has already declined and in a context of Western society where there is a limited timeframe to accomplish important life goals. The general population of women and potential age bankers in specific would benefit from campaigns creating more awareness on age related fertility decline and possible ways to counteract.

References

1. Stoop D, van der Veen F, Deneyer M, Nekkebroeck J, Tournaye H. Oocyte banking for anticipated gamete exhaustion (AGE) is a preventive intervention, neither social nor nonmedical. Reprod Biomed Online. 2014;28(5):548–51.
2. American Society for Reproductive Medicine (ASRM). ASRM urges caution, strong counseling for women seeking egg freezing; 2007. http://www.asrm.org/Media/Press/AM07urgecautioneggfreezing.html. Accessed 16 Oct 2007

3. Cutting R, Barlow S, Anderson R, On Behalf of ACE and BFS. Human oocyte cryopreservation: Evidence for practice. Hum Fertil. 2009;12(3):125–36. http://dx.doi.org/10.1080/14647270903132115. Published online 19 Sept 2009.
4. Harwood K. Egg freezing: a breakthrough for reproductive autonomy? Bioethics. 2009;23(1):39–46.
5. Goold A, Savulescu J. In favour of freezing for non-medical reasons. Bioethics. 2009;23(1):1467–8519.
6. Stoop D, Nekkebroeck J, Devroey P. A survey on the intentions and attitudes towards oocyte cryopreservation for non-medical reasons among women of reproductive age. Hum Reprod. 2011;26(3):655–61. doi:10.1093/humrep/deq367.
7. Sage CFF, Kolb BA, Treiser SL, Silverber KM, Barritt J, Copperman AB. Oocyte cryopreservation in women seeking elective fertility preservation: a multicentre analysis. Obstet Gynaecol. 2008;111:20S.
8. Ter Keurst A, Boivin J, Gameiro S. Women's intentions to use fertility preservation to prevent age-related fertility decline. Reprod Biomed Online. 2016;32:121–31.
9. Rogers E. Diffusion of innovations, 1st ed. Glencoe, UK: Free Press; (1962). In: Ter Keurst A, Boivin J, Gameiro S. Women's intentions to use fertility preservation to prevent age-relatied fertility decline. Reprod Biomed Online. 2016;32:121–31.
10. Mertes H, Pennings G. Social egg freezing: for better, not for worse. Reprod Biomed Online. 2011;23:824–9.
11. Gold E, Copperman K, Witkin G, Jones C, Copperman AB. A motivational assessment of women undergoing elective egg freezing for fertility preservation. Fertil Steril. 2006;86:S201. P-187
12. Baldwin K, Culley L, Hudson N, Mitchell H, Lavery S. Oocyte cryopreservation for social reasons: demographic and diposal intentions of UK users. Reprod Biomed Online. 2015;31:239–45.
13. Hodes-Wertz B, Druckenmiller S, Smith M, Noyes N. What do reproductive-age women who undergo oocyte cryopreservation think about the process as a means to preserve infertility? Fertil Steril. 2013;100(5):1343–9.
14. ESHRE Task Force on Ethics and Law, Dondorp W, de Wert G, Pennings G, Shenfield F, Devroey P, Tarlatzis B, Barri P, Diedrich K. Oocyte cryopreservation for age-related fertility loss. Hum Reprod. 2012;27(5):1231–7. doi:10.1093/humrep/des029.
15. Daniluk JC, Koert E. Childless women's beliefs and knowledge about oocyte freezing for social and medical reasons. Hum Reprod. 2016;31(10):2313–20. doi:10.1093/humrep/dew189.

Chapter 7
Ovarian Stimulation Prior to Elective Oocyte Cryopreservation

C. Iglesias and J.A. García-Velasco

Introduction

The demand of fertility preservation with no urgent medical indication or for social reasons has increased in recent years.

The main reason is that society has changed the traditional time for pregnancy for professional, personal or social reasons. Women decide to postpone their first pregnancy to a different time than when the biological fertile period is optimal.

Socio-cultural changes, longer life expectancy and professional activity have led to preserve fertility to guarantee the possibility of future pregnancy [1].

Gynecologists should perform the primary prevention of ovarian aging during gynecological reviews by measuring the ovarian follicle reserve and offering the oocyte freezing possibility.

Vitrification is an efficient method to preserve oocytes by quickly lowering temperature using liquid nitrogen (Chap. 8).

By this freezing method, cells are preserved and conserve the same characteristics and quality they had upon freezing [2] (Fig. 7.1).

Fertility preservation providers should inform women about their specific probabilities according to their age at vitrification, and emphasize the fact that egg freezing does not guarantee success, but increases the possibilities of having a biological child in the future [3].

Ovarian stimulation protocols should be as convenient, short and sure as possible to ease the procedure.

C. Iglesias, M.D. (✉) • J.A. García-Velasco, M.D.
IVI-Madrid, Rey Juan Carlos University,
Avenida del Talgo 68, Aravaca, Madrid 28023, Spain
e-mail: carlos.iglesias@ivi.es

© Springer International Publishing Switzerland 2018

D. Stoop (ed.), *Preventing Age Related Fertility Loss*,
DOI 10.1007/978-3-319-14857-1_7

	Vitrified	Fresh	P value
MII oocytes no. %	231 (87.2)	219 (89.7)	.363
MI oocytes no. %	19 (7.2)	11 (4.5)	.203
GV oocytes no. %	15 (5.7)	14 (5.7)	.974
Survival no. %	224/231 (96.9)	-	
No. Of injected oocytes	224	219	
Normal fertilization no. %	171 (76.3)	180 (82.2)	.128
Abnoraml fertilization no. %	9 (4%)	12 (5.4)	.469
Degenerated oocytes no. %	7 (3.1%)	6 (2.7)	.809

Fig. 7.1 Oocyte distribution, survival and fertilization (modified from Cobo A et al. Clinical outcome of oocyte vitrification. Fertil Steril. 2008)

Delaying the Desire of Pregnancy

Nowadays, more and more women contemplate the possibility of getting pregnant precisely when natural fertility is worse.

Various reasons justify society delaying the desire of pregnancy. In the last few years, economic problems have limited the possibility of emancipation and forming a family.

Women's professional activity makes it more difficult to deal with family conciliation issues and lack of time to attend its demands. Women in the western world are full-right city dwellers who adopt opposite attitudes to the traditional roles of domestic work and upbringing.

Longer life expectancy, facility of displacement, social activities and labor opportunities are other reasons to postpone first pregnancy [1].

This trend to leave first pregnancy until a later age and to a time when natural fertility is limited will diminish the possibility of getting pregnant.

Effect of Biological Aging on Ovarian Preservation

As time passes, the number of antral follicles begins to lower. This rhythm of progression is variable according to hereditary genetic determinants and environmental factors, like tobacco or exposure to environmental toxins and/or previous radio- or chemotherapy.

Initial publications by Menken, and more recently by Broekmans, have confirmed the progressive aging of ovarian reserve with time [4, 5] (Chap. 1).

This progressively slow deterioration begins at about the age of 30, and a more drastic quicker drop starts at around 35 years until ovarian reserve disappears in the first few years after reaching the age of 40.

This leads to higher oocyte aneuploidies, which reduce the quality of oocytes and, therefore, fertility.

Armstrong reported that advanced maternal age was related to meiotic incompetence, which makes fertilization rates rise by inducing anomalies in different embryonic development stages to induce more miscarriages.

Age-related abnormalities of oocytes include:

(a) meiotic incompetence or the inability to complete meiotic maturation, which results in oocytes being incapable of fertilization.
(b) errors in meiosis, which can be compatible with fertilization, but lead to genetic abnormalities that compromise embryo viability.
(c) cytoplasmic deficiencies, expressed in several development stages before or after fertilization [6]. Considering these effects of advanced age on oocyte quality, oocyte preservation should be performed as soon as possible to obtain more and better oocytes in women under the age of 35.

Evolution of Stimulation Protocols

The first IVF baby was born in a natural *in vitro* fertilization cycle without ovarian stimulation.

IVF success rates in natural cycles are low due to the limited number of oocytes retrieved per cycle. However, recent studies have shown that IVF in either a natural cycle or modified natural cycle might be a promising low-risk and low-cost alternative to standard stimulated IVF treatment since the available dominant follicle of each cycle is used [7].

Considering this limitation, ovarian stimulation initially using urinary gonadotropins significantly increases both the number of eggs retrieved and successful IVF rates.

In the natural cycle, follicular dominance is achieved by induced estradiol, which provides negative feedback to the pituitary gland which, in turn, lowers FSH levels.

In IVF stimulated cycles, addition of exogenous gonadotropins is used to achieve supra-threshold levels of gonadotropins in the follicular phase to induce multiple follicular recruitment.

However, various problems may occur in stimulated IVF cycles, like premature luteinization and failed synchronous follicular recruitment due to early dominant follicle selection, which implies lower success rates.

Another problem is spontaneous ovulation, which may occur at any time. So gonadotropin-releasing hormone agonists and antagonists (GnRHa and GnRHant) are used to induce pituitary desensitization in order to avoid spontaneous ovulation [8].

Pituitary desensitization using either GnRH agonists or GnRH antagonists eliminates possible interference by endogenous hormones, enables synchronous follicular development and prevents premature luteinization, which enhance the control oocyte retrieval of timing. Finally, the LH surge is substituted for exogenous hCG to induce oocyte retrieval [9].

Ovarian Stimulation Protocols for Oocyte Preservation

Different protocols have been proposed to hyperstimulate ovaries. Some protocols utilize GnRH agonists, while others use antagonists to achieve pituitary desensitization.

Protocols also vary as to the gonadotropins uemployed for ovarian stimulation, and recombinant or highly purified follicular stimulating hormone (rFSH or HP-FSH) are employed.

Addition of GnRH agonists to the luteal phase of the previous cycle in long protocols and in the early follicular phase in short protocols results in an initial flare-up effect, followed by pituitary desensitization.

In contrast, the GnRH antagonists (single or multiple doses) given in the mid-follicular phase, immediately prior to the rise in LH levels, results in rapid pituitary desensitization.

Long Protocol

This protocol starts in the mid-luteal phase of the previous cycle with GnRH agonists being administered daily for about 2 weeks or until down-regulation is completed.

Once down-regulation has been achieved, usually on the first days of menstruation, gonadotropins are administered subcutaneously to stimulate follicular growth with the GnRH agonist being continued at a lower dose.

The hMG/FSH dose is subsequently adjusted according to follicular growth, as monitored by serum E2 levels and transvaginal ultrasonography.

Human chorionic gonadotropin (hCG) is given once the follicular cohort consists of at least three follicles of over 18 mm in diameter to induce oocyte retrieval 36 h later.

This protocol provides excellent cycle control, but its longer treatment duration, higher gonadotropin consumption and more expensive cost are its main disadvantages.

There are different GnRH agonists, like buserelin, leuprorelin, nafarelin and triptorelin.

Nafarelin and buserelin can be administered as a nasal spray. They need to be given between twice and six times a day, and absorption fluctuates which results in an unpredictable response. However, buserelin, leuprorelin and triptorelin are administered as subcutaneous injections once a day.

Wong et al. published a meta-analyses of some trials by comparing different antagonist GnRH preparations. It found no difference in either pituitary suppression efficacy or IVF outcomes in terms of the number of oocytes collected and pregnancy rates. However, these authors reported that women treated with nafarelin required fewer ampoules of gonadotropins for ovarian stimulation, and fewer days of stimulation, compared to leuprorelin, triptorelin and buserelin.

The use of depot preparations of GnRH agonists has been associated with increased gonadotropin requirements and longer times for ovarian stimulation, even though IVF outcomes did not significantly differ [10].

Short Protocol Using GnRH Agonist

In this protocol, GnRH agonist administration starts in the early follicular phase and gonadotropins start the next day. Monitoring, hCG injection timing and oocyte retrieval are the same as with the long protocol.

This protocol in normally used for low-responder patients, or for those who presented a previous poor response in the long protocol, to obtain benefits from the initial flare-up of endogenous FSH release from the pituitary gland, which is induced on the first days of GnRH agonist administration [11].

Short Protocol Using GnRH Antagonist

GnRH antagonists are competitive inhibitors of endogenous GnRH given their receptor binding property, which rapidly inhibit gonadotropin secretion to reduce FSH and LH secretion within 8 h after administration, which is a potential advantage over GnRH agonists.

In this stimulation protocol, gonadotropins are administered on day 2 of the cycle and GnRH-ant is added in the mid-follicular phase to prevent premature LH surge.

Two different molecules, cetrorelix and ganirelix, are available, prove equally efficacious and can be used in two different protocols, the single and multiple dose protocols.

The multiple-dose GnRH-ant protocol involves daily subcutaneous injections of 0.25 mg of either cetrorelix or ganirelix from day 6 of stimulation (the fixed start) until the trigger administration of human chorionic gonadotropin (hCG) or the agonist trigger.

The single-dose protocol involves a single subcutaneous injection of 3 mg of GnRH-ant on day 7 or 8 of stimulation, which provides 4 days of pituitary suppression.

If the patient needs more days of stimulation, a daily dose of 0.25 mg of GnRH-ant injections is required until hCG trigger is performed. The monitoring, criteria for hCG administration and oocyte retrieval is similar to the agonist protocols.

In the flexible start protocol, addition of GnRH-ant begins when the diameter of the leading follicle is 14 mm or more.

In the multiple-dose GnRH-ant protocol daily subcutaneous injections of 0.25 mg of either cetrorelix or ganirelix are given until the trigger is performed.

However in the single-dose protocol, a single subcutaneous injection of 3 mg of GnRH-ant is injected when the diameter of the leading follicle is 14 mm or more to provide 4 days of pituitary suppression. If the patient needs more days of stimulation, daily 0.25-mg GnRH-ant injections are required until the trigger is performed. The monitoring criteria for hCG administration and oocyte retrieval are similar to the agonist protocols [12].

Fixed *Versus* flexible

Al-Inany et al. published a meta-analysis of randomized studies by comparing the fixed and flexible approaches. They concluded having found no statistically significant difference in pregnancy rates, despite finding a trend of the fixed protocol obtaining a higher pregnancy rate. However, the amount of the recombinant FSH and antagonist used with the flexible protocol significantly reduces [13].

Single *Versus* Multiple Dose GnRH Antagonist Protocol

The single dose GnRH antagonist protocol has the advantage of using fewer injections, with only 10% of cycles requiring additional daily doses of the GnRH antagonist.

The potential suppression of endogenous LH does not bring about any significant difference in pregnancy rates, as shown in a multicenter study that compared multiple and single dose protocols of cetrorelix [14].

Wilcox et al. published a prospective randomized trial, and found no significant difference in pregnancy rates between the ganirelix multiple dose and cetrorelix single dose protocols [15].

Advantages of the Antagonist Protocol

The antagonist protocol offers several advantages over the long one, which confirms the elective protocol in fertility preservation ovarian stimulation cycles. The advantages include: shorter treatment duration, fewer menopausal symptoms, less cyst formation due to the initial flare-up effect of GnRH, and fewer gonadotropin requirements.

	Mild protocol	GnRHant protocol	GnRH ag protocol	P value<0.05
Oocyte aspirations	166	1096	111	
FSH	6.4+-1.8	6.7+-2.1	6.9+-2	
Oocytes (per cycle)	1500(9+-5.2)	10249 (9.4+-5)	12004 (10.8+-5.6)	P=0.0001 (mild Vs antg P<0.0001(antg Vs ag)
MI oocytes %	240 (16)	1602 (15.6)	1687 (14.1)	P=0.0420 (mild Vs antg P<0.001(antg Vs ag)
2PN %	865 (57.7)	5440 (53.1)	6235 (51.9)	P=0.0009 (mild Vs ag P<0.0001(mild Vs ag)
Embryos%	845 (56.39)	5198 (50.7)	5968 (49.7)	P=0.0001 (mild Vs antg P<0.0001(mild Vs ag)
ET%	151 (91)	1017 (92.8)	1006 (90.5)	
Cycles with embryo freezing %	50 (30.1)	317 (28.9)	210 (18.9)	P=0.0008 (mild Vs ag P<0.0001(antg Vs ag)
OHHS	0	4	12	
Frozen embryos (per cylce)	0.8+-1.4	0.9+-1.8	0.5+-1.3	P=0.0243 (mild Vs ag P<0.0001(antg Vs ag)

Fig. 7.2 The COH outcome in terms of oocytes and embryos (modified from Stimpfel M et al. Comparison of GnRH agonist, GnRH antagonist, and GnRH antagonist mild protocol of controlled ovarian hyperstimulation in good prognosis patients. Int J Endocrinol. 2015)

Stimpfel et al. reported that the GnRH antagonist mild protocol of controlled ovarian stimulation could be the best method of choice in good prognosis patients due to significant differences in the average number of retrieved oocytes, immature oocytes, fertilized oocytes, embryos, transferred embryos, embryos frozen per cycle, and cycles with embryo freezing. However, this group did not identify any differences in live birth rates (LBR), miscarriages and ectopic pregnancies [12] (Figs. 7.2 and 7.3).

The most important advantage published in a Cochrane review is the significant reduction in the incidence of severe OHSS in antagonist cycles compared to agonist cycles ($p = 0.01$; $OR = 0.60$, 95%CI 0.40–0.88) [16].

Considering this information, in over-responders and polycystic ovarian syndrome patients, the GnRH-antagonist protocol lowered the incidence of OHSS in high responders.

The main advantage of this protocol is that the final oocyte maturation induced by the GnRH agonist can be used to prevent OHHS from developing [17] (Chap. 11).

	Mild protocol	Antagonist protocol	Agonist protocol	P value<0.05
Pregnancies	69	367	355	
P. Per cycle %	41.6	33.5	32	P=0.04 (mild Vs ang) P=0.01(mid Vs ag)
P per ET 23.2%22.1	45.7	36.1	35.3	P=0.02 (mild Vs antg) P=0.01(mid Vs ag)
Miscarriages %	23.2	22.1	19.4	
BQ preg	2	12	16	
LBR per cycle %	31.3	25.3	25.3	
LBR after FET	7	35	23	
Cumulative LBR per cycle %	35.6	28.5	27.3	P=0.02 (mild Vs antg)

Fig. 7.3 The outcome of COH in terms of pregnancies, miscarriages and deliveries (modified from Stimpfel M et al. Comparison of GnRH agonist, GnRH antagonist, and GnRH antagonist mild protocol of controlled ovarian hyperstimulation in good prognosis patients. Int J Endocrinol. 2015)

However, the antagonist cycle is less programmable than the agonist cycle, and such lack of flexibility poses a problem for some patients and IVF centers.

How to Optimize Ovarian Response

A normal response to ovarian stimulation is expected in patients aged under 40 with regular menstrual cycles (21–35 days), and a normal basal FSH (below 10), or normal AMH levels (2 ng/mL). This patient profile can be stimulated using both protocols to obtain similar results.

The response to stimulatory drugs in an IVF cycle depends on several factors: number of antral follicles, their sensitivity to FSH and bioavailability of FSH.

The expected response usually means the retrieval of 8–10 oocytes due to optimal ovarian stimulation.

Failure to recruit an adequate number of follicles and to retrieve 4–5 mature oocytes is termed a poor response, while the recruitment of 20 follicles or more in high responders increases the risk of OHSS.

To optimize ovarian response, personalization of protocols and selecting optimal gonadotropin doses should be considered.

The antagonist protocol should be offered to reduce the risk of ovarian hyperstimulation ovarian syndrome in patients with high ovarian reserves, like polycystic ovarian syndrome.

The flare-up protocol offers better success rates in women with low ovarian reserve as the long protocol leads to poor results in patients with poor ovarian reserve due to profound pituitary suppression.

Some models have been proposed to determine an optimal stimulation dose. Yet it is still difficult to obtain the desired response as ovarian response is affected by other factors that are yet to be determined [18].

Gonadotropin Dose Selection

Estimating the correct starting dose is extremely important to obtain optimal results.

A gonadotropin dose for standard patients varies between 100 and 250 IU/day.

However, ovarian response variability to the same gonadotropin is influenced by several factors that affect the response to controlled ovarian hyperstimulation, such as: patient's age, body mass index, smoking status, background of endometriosis, antral follicle count (AFC), ovarian volume, stromal blood flow, as well as endocrine parameters like basal FSH levels, inhibin B and Anti-Müllerian hormone serum levels.

The CONSORT study reported that the use of fixed dose regimens calculated by computerized dosing algorithms based on basal FSH, BMI, age and AFC resulted in adequate oocyte yield and good pregnancy rates (an overall of 34.2%) [19].

There are three gonadotropin dose regimes for ovarian stimulation:

- In the fixed dose regime, gonadotropin dose is kept constant throughout stimulation.
- In the step-down regime, a high starting dose of gonadotropins (300–450 IU) is used for the first 2 days, followed by a reduced dose (150–225 IU/day).
- This enables supra-physiological levels of gonadotropins to increase follicular recruitment in the early follicular phase and seems to result in greater follicle synchrony.
- In the step-up regime, the starting gonadotropin dose is low and is increased on cycle day 5, or later, depending on the response.

A variety of controlled ovarian stimulation protocols has been adopted with mixed success rates, but no single approach is appropriate for all patients in a given population. Treatment protocols should be adapted for individual patients to obtain as many oocytes as ovaries can produce. The more oocytes fertilized, the better chances of pregnancy patients will have (Fig. 7.4) [8].

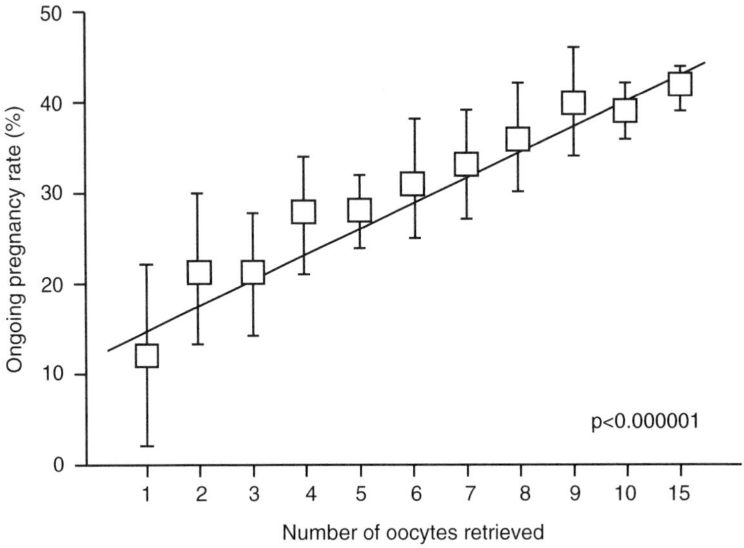

Fig. 7.4 (taken from Bosch E, Ezcurra D. Individualised controlled ovarian stimulation (iCOS): maximising success rates for assisted reproductive technology patients. Reprod Biol Endocrinol. 2011 Jun)

Ovarian Stimulation Cycle Control

Starting with spontaneous or induced menstruation, with previous birth control pill administration, an ultrasound scan should be done to confirm that both ovaries are inactive. Comparable outcomes can be obtained using an oral contraceptive pill that contains 0.030 mg of ethinyl estradiol and 0.15 mg of desogestrel to schedule the patients who undergo the antagonist protocol [20] (Fig. 7.5).

The ovarian stimulation period is variable with an average from 9 to 12 days of gonadotropin self-administration. Cycle monitoring is an essential part of any IVF protocol as it can indicate over- or under-response, which enables dose adjustments to optimize responses. This control is done by performing ultrasound scans every 2–3 days and measuring serum estradiol levels during stimulation.

One of the main aims of cycle monitoring is to prevent the ovarian over-response recognized during cycle monitoring. If the risk of OHSS seems very high, the final trigger is performed by an agonist trigger, and it also allows the next menstruation to start sooner due to the lutheolisis effect [21].

However, Kwan reported no significant difference in pregnancy rates and live births in the cycles monitored using ultrasound and serum estradiol, nor in those monitored by ultrasound alone [22].

The first monitoring visit is usually made on day 5 or 6 of stimulation when an ultrasound scan is done.

	OCP, n (%)	No OCP,n (%)	P value
BQ PR	61/115 (53)	67/113 (59.3)	.17
CPR	56/115 (48.7)	64/113 (56.6)	.12
OPR	55/115 (47.8)	61/113 (53.9)	.18
Multiple PR	15/56 (26.7)	18/64 (28.1)	.43
IR	75/207 (36.3)	80/204 (39.2)	.26
Miscarriage rate	5/56 (8.9)	11/64 (17)	.09
LBR	51/115 (44.3)	53/113 (47)	.35

Fig. 7.5 Cycle outcome (modified from García-Velasco et al. Cycle scheduling with OCPs. Fertil Steril. 2011)

The next scan control depends on ovarian response and is usually performed on day 8 or 9 of stimulation until follicles of 17 mm of diameter are measured and the final trigger is performed.

Random Start

Random start development in IVF cycles has taken huge strides to enable patients to vitrify oocytes when not much useful time is left.

In random-start protocols, the number of total and mature oocytes retrieved, oocyte maturity rate, mature oocyte yield and fertilization rates are similar to those in conventional (early follicular phase start) protocols.

When considering this approach, the random ovarian stimulation provides a main advantage as it shortens the total time for oocyte pick up, and ovarian stimulation in emergent settings can be started on a random cycle date for fertility preservation purposes without compromising oocyte yield and maturity [23].

Social Freezing Protocol at IVI Centers

The main stimulation protocol for social freezing that IVI centers use is the antagonist one with an agonist trigger.

This approach offers different advantages: fewer days of stimulation, patients do not need as many injections, and we can induce ovulation using a GnRHs agonist if a hyper-response of ovaries occurs. Finally, we can start a new stimulation sooner if the lutheal phase is shorter, if necessary.

We also consider administering long-acting FSH gonadotropins to avoid the daily pain of injections and to make stimulation easer for patients [24].

Considerations Before Treatment

It is important to inform patients properly about the procedure, and patients must deliver a signed informed consent with an explanation of the procedure, its risks and its success rates.

Patients should know that not all the antral follicles observed in the basal ultrasound scan will develop uniformly, not all follicles longer than 17 mm will have oocytes inside, and not all them will become mature oocytes that can be frozen.

Further relevant information that patients must receive is that the thawing rates of oocytes are higher than 90%, but they will depend on the patient's age and presence of some competing pathology that determines the quantity and quality of oocytes, such as the endometriosis, polycystic ovarian syndrome or previous ovarian surgery.

Patients should receive information about their chances of pregnancy depending on maternal age. Due to worse oocyte quality and a larger number of aneuploidies in patients older than 38, genetic preimplantation screening should be offered to select the euploid embryos to be transferred.

The aneuploid rate in patients aged between 38 and 42 years is 82–92%. The best practice in these patients is to reject aneuploid embryos and to select those with implantation possibilities.

Patients also should be informed about the commonest side effects during the procedure, like discomfort of injections in the place they are administered, morning sickness, headache and mood changes, the risks of anesthesia, injuries to pelvic organs, vaginal hemorrhage and post-surgery pain. These side effects are usually very mild and will have no long-term effects, regardless of the number of ovarian stimulation cycles [25].

One well-known complication is the risk of developing ovarian hyperstimulation syndrome. However, antagonists of GnRH stimulation protocols and the final trigger with GnRH agonist avoid this complication [2].

Patients should know that after oocyte pick up, menstruation will begin after 5–7 days. At this time, performing a scan of ovaries is recommended to determine their post-surgery status. If the number of retreived mature oocytes is lower than expected, a new ovarian stimulation can commence.

Key Messages

1. The election of the ovarian stimulation protocol as well as the gonadotropin doses based on AMH, BMI, age and AFC are crucial to optimize the ovarian response.
2. GnRH agonists or antagonists minimizes possible interferences by endogenous hormones, enables synchronous follicular development and prevents premature luteinization, which enhance the timing for oocyte retrieval.
3. The advantages of the antagonist protocol include shorter treatment duration and fewer gonadotropin requirements, fewer menopausal symptoms, lower cysts formation, and lower incidence of ovarian hyperstimulation syndrome.
4. Random start ovarian stimulation provides as main advantage the shortening of the interval from cycle initiation to oocyte pick up without compromising oocyte yield and maturity.
5. Long-acting FSH gonadotropins could be considered particularly in these patients to reduce the number of injections and to make stimulation protocols more convenient.

References

1. Birch Petersen K, et al. Family intentions and personal considerations on postponing childbearing in childless cohabiting and single women aged 35–43 seeking fertility assessment and counseling. Hum Reprod. 2015;30(11):2563–74.
2. Cobo A, et al. Oocyte vitrification as an efficient option for elective fertility preservation. Fertil Steril. 2016;105(3):755–64. e8
3. Cobo A, García-Velasco JA. Why all women should freeze their egg. Curr Opin Obstet Gynecol. 2016;28(3):206–10.
4. Menken J, Trussell J, Larsen U. Age and infertility. Science. 1986;234(5775):413.
5. FJM B, et al. Back to the basics of ovarian aging: a population-based study on longitudinal anti-Müllerian hormone decline. BMC Med. 2016;14(1):151.
6. Armstrong D. Effects of maternal age on oocyte developmental competence. Theriogenology. 2001;55(6):1303–22.
7. Allersma T, Farquhar C, Cantineau AE. Natural cycle in vitro fertilisation (IVF) for subfertile couples. Cochrane Database Syst Rev. 2013;30(8):CD010550. doi: 10.1002/14651858.CD010550.pub2.
8. Bosch E, Ezcurra D. Individualised controlled ovarian stimulation (iCOS): maximising success rates for assisted reproductive technology patients. Reprod Biol Endocrinol. 2011;9:82.
9. van Loendersloot LL, et al. Individualized decision-making in IVF: calculating the chances of pregnancy. Hum Reprod. 2013;28(11):2972–80.
10. Wong JM, Forrest KA, Snabes SZ, et al. Efficacy of nafarelin in assisted reproductive technology: a meta-analysis. Hum Reprod Update. 2001;7(1):92–101.
11. Pacchiarotti A, et al. Ovarian stimulation protocol in IVF: an up-to-date review of the literature. Curr Pharm Biotechnol. 2016;17(4):303–15.
12. Stimpfel M, et al. Comparison of GnRH agonist, GnRH antagonist, and GnRH antagonist mild protocol of controlled ovarian hyperstimulation in good prognosis patients. Int J Endocrinol. 2015;2015:385049.

13. Al-Inany HG, et al. Gonadotrophin-releasing hormone antagonists for assisted reproductive technology. Cochrane Database Syst Rev. 2016;4:CD001750.
14. Olivennes F, et al. Multiple Dose International Study Group.; Cetrotide Single Dose International Study Group. Safety and efficacy of a 3 mg dose of the GnRH antagonist cetrorelix in preventing premature LH surges: report of two large multicentre, multinational, phase IIIb clinical experiences. Reprod Biomed Online. 2003;6(4):432–8.
15. Wilcox J, et al. Prospective, randomized trial comparing cetrorelix acetate and ganirelix acetate in a programmed, flexible protocol for premature luteinizing hormone surge prevention in assisted reproductive technologies. Fertil Steril. 2005;84(1):108–17.
16. Al-Inany HG, Abou-Setta AM, Aboulghar M. Gonadotrophin-releasing hormone antagonists for assisted conception: a Cochrane review. Reprod Biomed Online. 2007;14(5):640–9.
17. Krishna D, Dhoble S, Praneesh G, Rathore S, Upadhaya A, Rao K. Gonadotropin-releasing hormone agonist trigger is a better alternative than human chorionic gonadotropin in PCOS undergoing IVF cycles for an OHSS Free Clinic: A Randomized control trial. J Hum Reprod Sci. 2016;9(3):164–72.
18. Popovic-Todorovic B, Loft A, Lindhard A, Bangsbøll S, Andersson AM, Andersen AN. A prospective study of predictive factors of ovarian response in 'standard' IVF/ICSI patients treated with recombinant FSH. A suggestion for a recombinant FSH dosage normogram. Hum Reprod. 2003;18(4):781–7.
19. Pouly JL, French CONSORT Study Group, et al. Usability and utility of the CONSORT calculator for FSH starting doses: a prospective observational study. Reprod Biomed Online. 2015;31(3):347–55.
20. Garcia-Velasco JA, et al. Cycle scheduling with oral contraceptive pills in the GnRH antagonist protocol vs the long protocol: a randomized, controlled trial. Fertil Steril. 2011;96(3):590–3. doi:10.1016/j.fertnstert.2011.06.022.
21. Banker M, Garcia-Velasco JA. Revisiting ovarian hyper stimulation syndrome: Towards OHSS free clinic. J Hum Reprod Sci. 2015;8(1):13–7. doi:10.4103/0974-1208.153120. Review.
22. Kwan I, Bhattacharya S, Kang A, Woolner A. Monitoring of stimulated cycles in assisted reproduction (IVF and ICSI). Cochrane Database Syst Rev. 2014;24(8):CD005289. doi: 10.1002/14651858.CD005289.pub3.
23. Cakmak H, Rosen MP. Random-start ovarian stimulation in patients with cancer. Curr Opin Obstet Gynecol. 2015;27(3):215–21.
24. Requena A, et al. Evaluation of the degree of satisfaction in oocyte donors using sustained-release FSH corifollitropin α. Reprod Biomed Online. 2013;26(3):253–9.
25. Fatemi HM, et al. Severe ovarian hyperstimulation syndrome after gonadotropin-releasing hormone (GnRH) agonist trigger and "freeze-all" approach in GnRH antagonist protocol. Fertil Steril. 2014;101(4):1008–11.

Chapter 8
Oocyte Cryopreservation Technique

Neelke De Munck, Gábor Vajta, and Laura Rienzi

Introduction

Cryopreservation of human oocytes can be performed by both slow freezing and vitrification. In 1986, the first report of a pregnancy from frozen-thawed oocytes was obtained [1]. Since this report, many efforts were made to improve the efficiency of the cryopreservation protocols, both for slow-freezing and vitrification. It was more than one decade later that a live birth was described after oocyte vitrification [2] and it was only in 2005 that a highly efficient and reproducible vitrification protocol for human oocytes was obtained [3]. Both methods are currently still applied although the results obtained with vitrification appear to be superior to the ones obtained with slow-freezing [4].

Indications for Oocyte Cryopreservation

Tremendous increases obtained regarding oocyte survival and clinical pregnancy rates during the last decade led to a widespread application of this technique for many indications. While in the beginning this technique was mainly used in oocyte donation programmes—eliminating the problem of donor-recipient synchronization

N. De Munck (✉)
Centre for Reproductive Medicine, Laarbeeklaan 101, 1090 Brussels, Belgium
e-mail: neelke.demunck@uzbrussel.be

G. Vajta
Central Queensland University, Bruce Highway, North Rockhampton, QLD, Australia

L. Rienzi
GENERA Center for Reproductive Medicine,
Clincia Valle Giulia, via de notaris 2b, Rome, Italy

© Springer International Publishing Switzerland 2018

D. Stoop (ed.), *Preventing Age Related Fertility Loss*,
DOI 10.1007/978-3-319-14857-1_8

and allowing an efficient distribution of oocytes among different recipients—its use could also be beneficial in medical and non-medical fertility preservation programmes.

Women diagnosed with malignant diseases have the opportunity to vitrify oocytes before their gonadotoxic treatment. Depending on how fast the treatment should start and on the hormone receptivity of the tumor, fertility preservation for these patients may be obtained by vitrifying mature oocytes after controlled ovarian stimulation (COS), after *in vitro* maturation (IVM), or after *ex vivo* IVM. In the latter technique, very often used in prepubertal children in combination with ovarian tissue cryopreservation, IVM is performed on immature oocytes retrieved from the extracorporeal ovarian tissue after ovariectomy. Patients with some non-oncological medical conditions including genetic predisposition for premature ovarian failure or endometriosis could also benefit from oocyte vitrification. Finally, women postponing childbirth because of personal ambitions or lack of a partner have the opportunity to vitrify oocytes at a younger age and use them later on if they are confronted with age-related fertility loss.

The Oocyte

By the time the oocyte ovulates, some major oocyte maturation processes have taken place; these include both nuclear and cytoplasmic maturation during which the oocyte grows in size [5]. Nuclear maturation involves completion of the first meiotic division leading to extrusion of the first polar body and initiation of the second meiotic division with an arrest in metaphase II stage of meiosis [6]. Cytoplasmic maturation is indispensable to acquire an oocyte with a high developmental potency; it includes proper spatial and temporal reorganization and redistribution of the cytoplasmic organelles (mitochondria (M), Golgi apparatus, smooth endoplasmic reticulum (SER) and cortical granules) and the cytoskeleton.

Since the oocyte has a specific nuclear and cytoplasmic arrangement, important to achieve fertilization and adequate development, the structural and functional integrity should be maintained during vitrification. However, by exposing the oocyte to the highly concentrated cryoprotective additives (CPAs; often mentioned also as cryoprotectants) some physical and chemical parameters, e.g. osmotic pressure, pH, ionic intracellular content) fluctuate over a wide non-physiological range which may impact structural and genomic integrity [7]. Besides, this exposure also leads to osmotic stress and the repeated volumetric changes may result in a significant loss of functional integrity and even cell death [8]. In order to maintain this integrity during vitrification, a perfect interplay should be applied between (1) cooling and warming rate, (2) CPA choice and their concentration and working temperature, (3) the device and the minimal volume that they allow to load.

This interplay should also take into account the biological variability between oocytes. Different oocytes, even from the same patient, may react differently upon exposure to hyperosmotic solutions. These differences in permeability and inactive volume have been attributed to inherent biological variability [9, 10]. Besides this, the use of different stimulation protocols in assisted reproductive technology (ART) may influence the biological variability even more. The high variations in membrane permeability between oocytes make it hard to establish a fixed highly reproducible cryopreservation protocol. Even if a theoretical model would be established using the mean permeability coefficients, it would be sub-optimal for a number of oocytes. Therefore, a more robust protocol, eliminating the effects of the biological variability may deviate from the theoretical optimal protocol.

Ultrastructure

Since the oocyte is the starting point of a new life, the oocyte vitrification procedure should not induce ultrastructural changes that may affect further developmental competence nor health of the liveborn. While immediate survival can be observed by light microscopy, this will not show the ultrastructural changes of the spindle or the cytoplasmic organelles. The spindle is mainly analyzed by confocal microscopy or by Polscope analysis before and after warming. Polscope analysis showed a high spindle re-appearance, both after open or closed oocyte vitrification while confocal microscopy showed comparable results to fresh oocytes [11, 12] or a compromised chromosome alignment [13]. The following differences are observed when fresh and vitrified oocytes are compared by electron microscopy: a slightly higher vacuolization, smaller M-SER complexes, a decrease or abnormality in the microvillar structure and a decrease in the amount and density of the cortical granules [14–17]. When these features are compared between open or closed vitrification devices, the ultrastructure is better preserved in open devices [18]. Besides this, a reduced ATP production in open devices [19] and losses and alterations in the mRNA content in open and closed devices have been observed [20, 21].

These subtle differences between fresh and vitrified oocytes may have consequences for further development. Displacement of the spindle (Fig. 8.1) may result in the potential disturbance in alignment of chromosomes and ultimately aneuploidy [22]. Abnormalities in the mitochondria or M-SER complexes (Fig. 8.2) lead to reduced fertilization potential due to disturbances in Ca^{2+} homeostasis. The increased number of vacuoles (Fig. 8.3) is thought to be responsible for an inward organelle displacement which might have further negative developmental consequences [23]. Finally, the reduction in cortical granules, probably due to the premature release of their content leading to zona hardening, together with the altered microvillar

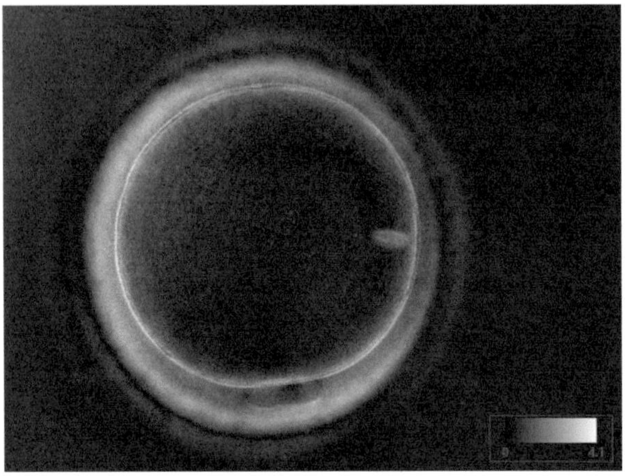

Fig. 8.1 MII human oocyte showing meiotic spindle displacement after warming

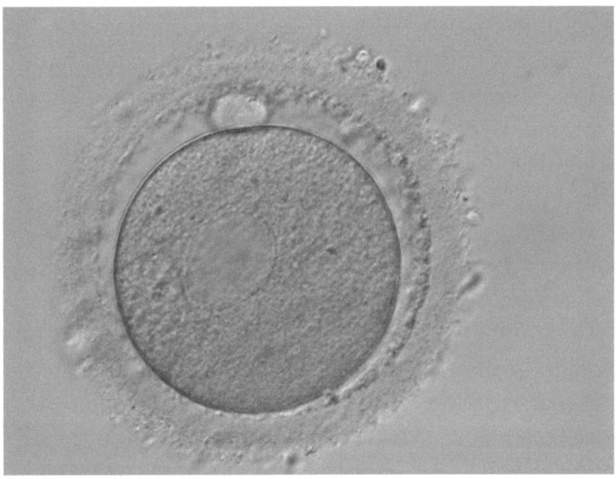

Fig. 8.2 MII human oocyte displaying M-SER complexes

structure leads to an ineffective oocyte-spermatozoon fusion. These differences between fresh and vitrified oocytes and their impact on further development have not only been described in human oocytes, but also in other species [24–26].

Knowing the high successes obtained to date, it is clear that the oocyte tolerates some of the ultrastructural changes induced by the vitrification procedure. However, due to the small number of studies comparing open and closed devices, it is still unclear whether the increased ultrastructural changes observed in closed devices also have a more pronounced effect on the developmental competence and clinical outcomes.

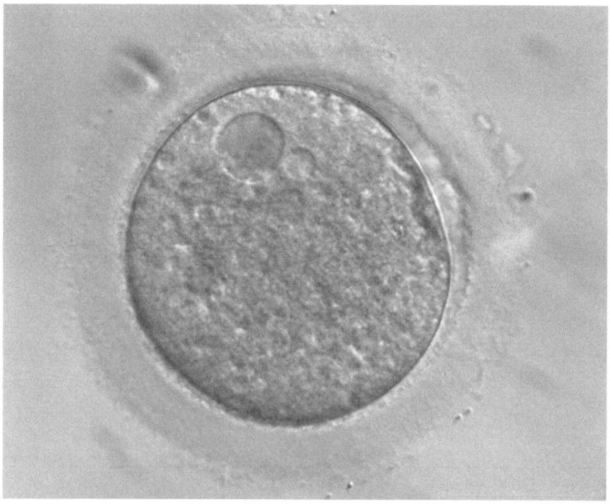

Fig. 8.3 Increased vacuolization in vitrified/warmed oocyte

Biophysical Properties

To be able to understand the volumetric changes of an oocyte upon exposure to one or more CPAs at different temperatures, several biophysical properties should be taken into account [27]. The practical use, however, should also take into account other parameters like the biological variability between oocytes and the CPA toxicity.

The *hydraulic conductivity* (L_p) or the permeability of the oocyte to water is the flow of water across each unit of the cell surface as a function of time. When an oocyte is exposed to an extracellular hypertonic solution, the initial response will be a relatively fast shrinkage because water leaves the cell. This initial volume reduction in a short time period will mainly determine L_p [28] and depends on the type and the concentration of the CPA and the exposure temperature. This volume reduction is followed by a gradual entering of the CPA in the oocyte to return to a volume slightly greater than the initial isotonic volume. This re-expansion determines the *solute permeability* (L_{CPA}) or the permeability of the oocyte to CPAs. CPAs with a high permeability will be loaded in the cell more quickly. Therefore the total volume excursion experienced by the cell will be reduced. A higher exposure temperature leads to a less extensive shrinkage/swelling response and reduces consequently the osmotic stress. This higher temperature will unfortunately also increase the unbeneficial effects of CPAs' toxicity [10].

The *activation energy* (E_A) or the temperature dependence of L_p and L_{CPA} [29] gives the minimal amount of energy that is needed to transport water or other molecules through the cell membrane. The lower the activation energy, the faster the molecules move across the cell membrane. By plotting the values for the hydraulic and solute permeability (Y-axis) at the different temperatures (X-axis), the activation energy (E_A) is indicated by the slope: $E_A = -R*slope$; R = gas constant.

The *inactive volume* (V_b) or the part of the oocyte's volume that is osmotically inactive is defined by exposing the oocyte to a non-permeating hyperosmotic solution. For mature human oocytes this is around 20% of the iso-osmotic volume [30].

The *surface-to-volume ratio* of the oocyte: since the spherical human oocyte has a large diameter, the surface-to-volume ratio is very low. This makes oocytes less efficient in losing water and taking up CPAs. Therefore, oocytes are more susceptible to cryodamage if the exposure to CPAs is not long enough. It is, together with the osmotic inactive volume, an important factor related to the formation of lethal intracellular ice during freezing [31].

The importance of these properties can be summarized as follows: (1) the oocyte has a different membrane permeability for water and individual CPAs which is highly temperature dependent, (2) oocytes cannot shrink to less than 20% of their original volume, (3) oocytes need a long exposure time to CPAs because of their big spherical shape and (4) oocytes will not re-expand to their original volume if they are exposed to partially permeable CPAs.

Vitrification

Principles

The cryobiological definition of vitrification is ice-free amorphous solidification of both intra- and extracellular solutions at subzero temperatures [32]. It can also be regarded as an extremely increased viscosity of these solutions [33]. To induce this phenomenon, special circumstances are required, such as increased cooling rates, and high concentrations of CPAs. However, neither rapid cooling, nor CPAs are indispensable factors: pure water can also be vitrified when extremely rapid cooling rates are applied and vitrification also occurs at low cooling rates when highly concentrated CPAs are used. On the other hand, extremely high cooling rates are difficult to obtain under average embryology laboratory circumstances; and the toxic and osmotic effect of highly concentrated CPAs required for vitrification at slow cooling rates may be detrimental to the biological sample [34]. Accordingly a delicate balance between these two factors is used in current vitrification protocols.

It should also be noted that approaches to prevent ice-crystal induced damage are very similar in both traditional slow-rate freezing and vitrification. Both processes are based on a stepwise increase of permeable and non-permeable CPAs to induce dehydration and a high intra- and pericellular permeable CPA concentration. During slow-rate freezing, this increase is obtained by applying a controlled slow cooling rate, leading to the formation of extracellular ice that will further dehydrate the cell. When the cell is dehydrated before the temperature of intracellular ice formation is reached, an ice-free solidification in and around the sample occurs. On the other hand, in most vitrification protocols, samples are exposed to increasing CPA solutions at room temperature or at the body temperature of the mammalian species. When samples are subsequently cooled rapidly, the whole solution will solidify without ice formation [35].

Theoretically, both processes can be successful. In practice—and in spite of the low level of standardization and lack of automation that may cause considerable inter-operator variability—vitrification seems to result in more consistent and higher survival and subsequent developmental rates [4]. Also, vitrification is the approach used in most human IVF laboratories for oocyte cryopreservation. Accordingly, the rest of this chapter will focus on vitrification.

Exposure to CPAs

The role of CPAs is crucial in cryopreservation of mammalian cells and tissues since their major function is to guard cells from cryodamage. Dozens of materials were tested, but only a handful was selected, mostly empirically, some of them entirely by chance. CPAs are commonly divided into two categories, permeable and non-permeable ones.

Theoretically, the role of permeable CPAs is to enter cells and replace a considerable amount of the intracellular water. This simple exchange may decrease the amount of ice formed; an additional effect of these materials is a more complex molecular mechanism that may vary between various CPAs. The final intracellular concentration of permeable CPAs may be rather high, therefore the level of toxicity is an important factor when selecting the right material. It should be noted, however, that the mechanism and tolerance level of toxic effect for cells, including oocytes and embryos, may be different of those for complex organs. Isolated cells may survive with an order of magnitude higher concentrations of permeable CPAs than living mammalian organisms.

Permeable CPAs commonly used for vitrification—selected purely on an empirical basis, –are organic solvents including ethylene glycol (EG), dimethyl sulphoxide (DMSO) and propylene glycol (PG). Since they are characterized by a low molecular weight, these molecules easily penetrate cell membranes. Glycerol, that has resulted in an unexpected breakthrough in sperm cryopreservation in the early 50s was found suboptimal for vitrification. EG, a major component of car coolants was a logical choice and its applicability is widely accepted in embryology (in sharp contrast with its potentially fatal nephrotoxicity). On the other hand, there is an ethernal debate between reproductive cryobiologist between DMSO and PG. Some companies advertise their DMSO-free CPA solutions as "non-toxic", although this statement is rather controversial; PG, that is used for replacement may have higher toxic and mutagenic effect than DMSO itself (reviewed in [36]).

In fact, except for a very early experiment, no late (*in vivo*) pathological consequences of CPA exposure during vitrification were detected, and today's commonly used techniques have successfully decreased the required concentration and use two permeable CPAs instead of one to minimize the specific toxic effect of both of them. Accordingly the main point of selection is the efficiency and not the imaginary toxicity. The majority of published works describing high survival and subsequent *in vitro—in vivo* developmental rates use 50–50% combination of EG and DMSO as permeable CPAs, respectively.

For non-permeable CPAs, their role is to provide a relatively neutral osmotic pressure to expell intracellular water to close of the maximum tolerable level. Different forms of sugars were tested. In early vitrification protocols, Ficoll was a common component, later on replaced by the common sugar, sucrose (saccharose) or trehalose. Although several publications suggest the use of trehalose, no conclusive evidence supports its superiority, and sucrose has remained the most common component of CPA solutions [35].

Although rarely discussed, the role of basic (holding) media cannot be neglected, either. Successful vitrification can be performed by using the simplest buffers including PBS, but more complex media may provide more consistent outcomes. According to our experience TCM-199, one of the most complex media (that has been replaced decades ago by simpler and more appropriate solutions for embryo culture) is uniquely suitable for vitrification purposes. The Hepes-buffered version—in contrast to other buffers—was also found to be more stabile during storage at 4 °C, minimising one factor that may lead to inconsistent outcomes. Supplementation of basic media with biopolymers also seems to be beneficial for survival of cryodamage. The most complex blood serum was a previously indispensable component of vitrification solutions in rather high concentrations. Due to legal restrictions motivated by potential disease transmission and toxicity issues, it has been subsequently replaced with human serum albumin or—preferably—preparations containing both albumin and globulin. Recently, a semisynthetic water soluble polymer hydroxypropil cellulose was suggested to replace blood proteins to further minimize inconsistencies [37], but the conclusive evidence of its superiority is still missing. All these biopolymers may have stabilizing effects on cellular membranes, although the exact mechanism still requires further clarification. It should also be noted that addition of antifreeze proteins, that are part of the surviving strategy of some vertebrates on cold climates, did not fulfill the—otherwise quite resonable—expectations.

Addition of CPAs is usually a stepwise process, with minimum two steps involved (Fig. 8.4). The two steps have two different functions in the protection strategy, even if these differences are slightly overlapping and not realized by most operators. The first step includes equilibration with a relatively low concentration of permeable CPAs (usually half of the final amount), and without addition of non-permeable ones. The relatively short (around 3 min) equilibration phase applied in earlier methods was replaced with rather long (10–21 min) equilibration improving considerably the outcome [38]. For large and osmotically sensitive biological samples including human oocytes, the initial phase of exposition is further distributed to several steps, resulting in a semilinear increase of CPAs. Oocytes are supposed to regain their original shape after each phase; in fact—as the rate of equilibration may depend on the individual physico-chemical characteristics of oocytes—the full

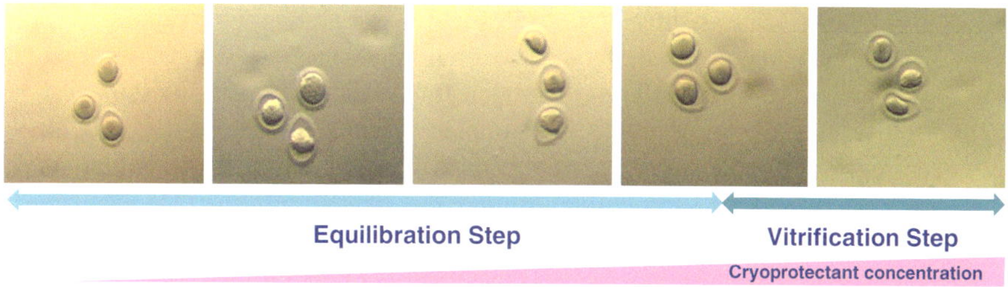

Fig. 8.4 Human oocyte vitrification procedure: the stepwise addition of CPA allows for a gradual dehydration of oocytes. Before exposure to the vitrification solution, oocytes are supposed to regain their original shape

length of the process should be adjusted to the microscopic picture [3]. The recovery of the intracellular volume means that an approximate equilibrium of CPAs and water was achieved between the intra- and extracellular space, respectively. However, this concentration of CPAs is insufficient to protect extra- and intracellular solutions from ice formation. It is only the second step, the exposition of the concentrated CPA solution that will ensure conditions required for ice-free solidification. In this step, ocytes/embryos are exposed to highly concentrated permeable CPAs (15–16% v/v) and approx. 1 M sucrose. This exposition has to be rapid (usually less than 1 min), and aggressive, with vigorous mixing and pipetting. During this short period, only a small amount of permeable CPAs enters the cytoplasm, the rest just contributes in the strong osmotic pressure established together with the high sucrose concentration. As the result of this joint effect, the ball turns into a disc or even more frequently half of it folds into the other half, and the maximum tolerable amount of water leaves the cell. This is the moment when a rapid cooling is required.

Cooling and Warming Rates

According to the empirically established parameters, safe cooling and warming rates for embryological samples should be above 20,000 °C/min for vitrification and warming [39]. Although some publications suggest that lower cooling rates do not compromise efficiency, the experimental basis of these attempts has been established in mouse oocytes that are rather tolerant to cryodamage(s), and developmental competence was not investigated [40–42]. A few recent papers dealing with human oocyte vitrification also argue that cooling rates are less critical [43–45]. However, according to the experience of authors of this paper—and probably thousands of laboratories worldwide—decreased cooling rates may lead to decreased consistency and compromised outcomes.

Submerging samples in liquid nitrogen is the standard and relatively easily available approach for cooling and storage to/at low temperatures. Liquefied forms of other gasses may offer slightly higher rates and lower storage temperatures, but—due to problems with availability and price, their application is extremely restricted. On the other hand, exposing liquid nitrogen to vacuum decreases its temperature below the standard boiling point, and samples immersed into this "supercooled" liquid nitrogen will cool more rapidly, in lack of a thermo-insulating vapour coat that develops around the sample upon immersion. This option may have considerable perspectives, unfortunately the exploitation is slower than expected.

Most research in the past 20 years has been focused to optimize the sample size and to minimize its insulation. Obviously, a smaller sample may ensure higher cooling and warming rates. Small samples may also decrease the danger of heterogenous ice nucleation, formation of small spots of ice inside the sample [46]. Simple dropping of samples into liquid nitrogen was not found practical, and cooling rates remained relatively high, as these drops were floating on the surface for seconds, due to the evaporation of the liquid nitrogen beneath. Carrier tools obtained from other fields of biology or specially developed for this purpose and holding (preferably) less than 1 μL solution were required. A summary of these tools has been provided earlier [34, 35] and their benefits and disadvantages will be also discussed at the end of this chapter.

With an appropriate carrier tool, warming is a simple task. In optimal systems, vitrified samples are immersed directly into the medium pre-warmed to the core temperature of the mammal. Usually samples may get separated spontaneously from the carrier tool shortly after immersion, and may be processed alone subsequently.

Removal of Cryoprotectants

Direct rehydration, i.e. transferring cryopreserved samples from liquid nitrogen directly into the holding medium without any osmotic buffer is an option for certain embryos after some special slow-rate freezing techniques, and was also applied successfully after vitrification of bovine embryos. However, this approach may be risky for human embryos, and is definitely detrimental for human oocytes. To prevent extreme swelling and lysis, the high intracellular osmotic pressure must be counterbalanced by an osmotic buffer consisting of the concentrated solution of the non-permeable CPA applied for vitrification, i.e. in most cases sucrose or trehalose. The concentration of the osmotic buffer may be carefully decreased in two or three steps. One or two thorough washes in the holding medium are followed by incubation in maturation medium, then ICSI.

Devices

In the initial period, vitrification was performed in 0.25 mL straws or cryovials developed for slow-rate freezing in embryology or cell-tissue culture, respectively. Subsequently, to decrease the volume to the required level various devices obtained from other fields of science were used including electron microscopic grids [47]. The open pulled straw (OPS) was the first device developed for embryo/oocyte vitrificationpurposes [39] followed by other tools including the Cryotop, Cryotip, Cryoleaf, Cryohook, etc. (see reviewed in [34, 35]). In a short period, almost every scientist working in reproductive cryobiology has developed his own method, and faced troubles not only in proving its superiority over the previous ones, but also in finding a relevant name. Eventually about a dozen of different devices remained and reached the level of commercial production. These devices are commonly sorted into two groups. In the first group, samples are exposed directly to the cooling and warming solutions allowing the highest possible cooling and warming rates, but the lack of a barrier layer means a potential danger of contamination from the infected liquid nitrogen [48]. In the other group, samples are isolated from liquid nitrogen, decreasing both the cooling rate and the danger of contamination. It has to be clarified whether some of the so-called closed devices are either not safely closed or result in a compromised situation at warming. The problem including the possible consequences has been discussed in detail in a recent review [49].

In some areas of reproductive biology, the cooling rate provided by several closed devices may be satisfactory. However, for human samples, especially human oocytes the compromised cooling rate may be insufficient. While inventors and producers of certain closed devices emphasize their superiority, the number of relevant publications is still insufficient to talk about conclusive evidence(s). On the other hand, the vast majority of groups continued to use the highly successful open devices for oocyte vitrification, in spite of the existing or potential legal restrictions. After more than a million of babies and several million of transfers after vitrification in open devices, without a single documented case of infection caused by liquid nitrogen mediated disease transmission, professional and legal authorities are more or less convinced not to interfere and let one of the most successful inventions in human embryology be applied properly. On the other hand, inventors, producers and clinics have implemented measures to minimize even the theoretical danger, using sterile containers for storage and/or contamination free liquid nitrogen for cooling [50–52].

Standardization, Safety and Automation

Due to various devices, CPAs and parameters, vitrification in human reproduction cannot be considered as a method or technique, it is rather an approach with some common principles but extremely diverse realization. Moreover, the rapid spreading of methods all over the world has resulted in an inappropriate education and application. Manuals and videos without personal teaching are insufficient; personal teaching without a qualified instructor, performed by poorly informed marketing agents and recently involved colleagues may be inadequate. Hands-on vitrification workshops are held worldwide, but offer access only to a limited number of embryologists, and many of them serve predominantly marketing and not educational purposes. Accordingly, results achieved in an average clinic may be below the expectations and the intrinsic capability of the given technology.

Moreover, vitrification in embryology is performed by the alternative use of the microscopes, delicate micropipetting and the liquid nitrogen placed in open containers close to the operator. Strict safety rules determine the required clothes, gloves and protective glasses while working with liquid nitrogen. Practically none of them are, and very few of them can be followed in the routine process of embryo/oocyte vitrification. The situation was more or less tolerable in a research laboratory where ad hoc solutions are common, but vitrification is now part of the everyday practice in any reproductive laboratory, with staff improperly informed about potential hazards.

As vitrification is now a key element of human assisted reproduction, to resolve problems related to standardization and work safety is indispensable. It should also be realized that all actually used manual vitrification techniques are extremely primitive. There are attempts to change this situation by introducing devices that are capable to automate some isolated phases of the process. However, future directions should focus on more complex and more intelligent solutions including machines capable to perform both equilibration and cooling, or both warming and dilution, respectively. This advancement may require a significant investment including intellectual input and financial support.

However, considering the past achievements and the future perspectives, the required investment does not seem to be disproportional.

Key Message

1. Oocyte vitrification affects the oocyte ultrastructure
2. High cooling and warming rates are a pre-requisite
3. No contamination has been observed when using open devices
4. Safe, standardized, automated vitrification systems may become a reality.

References

1. Chen C. Pregnancy after human oocyte cryopreservation. Lancet. 1986;1(8486):884–6.
2. Kuleshova L, Gianaroli L, Magli C, Ferraretti A, Trounson A. Birth following vitrification of a small number of oocytes: a case report. Hum Reprod. 1999;14(12):3077–9.
3. Kuwayama M, Vajta G, Kato O, Leibo SP. Highly efficient vitrification method for cryopreservation of human oocytes. Reprod Biomed Online. 2005;11(3):300–8.
4. Paramanantham J, Talmor A, Osianlis T, Weston GC. Cryopreserved oocytes: update on clinical applications and success rates. Obstet Gynecol Surv. 2015;70:97–114.
5. Guraya SS. Cellular and molecular biology of human oogenesis, ovulation and early embryogenesis. New Delhi: New Age International Publishers; 2008.
6. Seidler GE. Mammalian oocytes and preimlantation embryos as methodological components. Biol Reprod. 1983;28:36–49.
7. Kopeika J, Thornhill A, Khalaf Y. The effect of cryopreservation on the genome of gametes and embryos: principles of cryobiology and critical appraisal of the evidence. Hum Reprod Update. 2015;21(2):209–17.
8. Chen SU, Lien YR, Chao KH, Ho HN, Yang YS, Lee TY. Effects of cryopreservation on meiotic spindles of oocytes and its dynamics after thawing: clinical implications on oocyte freezing-a review article. Mol Cell Endocrinol. 2003;202(1–2):101.7.

9. Hunter J, Bernard A, Fuller B, McGrath J, Shaw RW. Plasma membrane water permeabilities of human oocytes: the temperature dependence of water movement in individual cells. J Cell Physiol. 1992;150(1):175–9.
10. Paynter SJ. A rational approach to oocyte cryopreservation. Reprod Biomed Online. 2005;10(5):578–86.
11. Cobo A, Pérez S, De los Santos MJ, Zulategui J, Domingo J, Remohí J. Effect of different cryopreservation protocols on the metaphase II spindle in human oocytes. Reprod Biomed Online. 2008;17(3):350–9.
12. Cao YX, Xing Q, Li L, Cong L, Zhang ZG, Wei ZL, Zhou P. Comparison of survival and embryonic development in human oocytes cryopreserved by slow-freezing and vitrification. Fertil Steril. 2009;92(4):1306–11.
13. Coticchio G, Bromfield JJ, Sciajno R, Gambardella A, Scaravelli G, Borini A, Albertini DF. Vitrification may increase the rate of chromosome misalignment in the metaphase II spindle of human mature oocytes. Reprod Biomed Online. 2009;19(Suppl 3):29–34.
14. Nottola SA, Coticchio G, Sciajno R, Gambardella A, Maione M, Scaravelli G, Bianchi S, Macchiarelli G, Borini A. Ultrastructural markers of quality in human mature oocytes vitrified using cryoleaf and cryoloop. Reprod Biomed Online. 2009;19(Suppl 3):17–27.
15. Gualtieri R, Mollo V, Barbato V, Fiorentino I, Iaccarino M, Talevi R. Ultrastructure and intracellular calcium response during activation in vitrified and slow-frozen human oocytes. Hum Reprod. 2011;26(9):2452–60.
16. Bianchi V, Macchiarelli G, Borini A, Lappi M, Cecconi S, Miglietta S, Familiari G, Nottola SA. Fine morphological assessment of quality of human mature oocytes after slow freesing or vitrification with a closed device: a comparative analysis. Reprod Biol Endocrinol. 2014;12:110.
17. Palmerini MG, Antinori M, Maione M, Cerusico F, Versaci C, Nottola SA, Macchiarelli G, Khalili MA, Antinori S. Ultrastructure of immature and mature human oocytes after cryotop vitrification. J Reprod Dev. 2014;60(6):411–20.
18. Bonetti A, Cervi M, Tomei F, Marchini M, Ortolani F, Manno M. Ultrastructural evaluation of human metaphase II oocytes after vitrification: closed versus open devices. Fertil Steril. 2011;95(3):928–35.
19. Manipalviratn S, Tong ZB, Stegmann B, Wildra E, Carter J, DeCherney A. Effect of vitrification and thawing on human oocyte ATP concentration. Fertil Steril. 2011;95(5):1839–41.
20. Chamayou S, Bonaventura G, Alecci C, Tibullo D, Di Raimondo F, Guglielmino A, Barcellona ML. Consequences of metaphase II oocyte cryopreservation on mRNA content. Cryobiology. 2011;62(2):130–4.
21. Monzo C, Haouzi D, Roman K, Assou S, Dechaud H, Hamamah S. Slow freezing and vitrification differentially modify the gene expression profile of human metaphase II oocytes. Hum Reprod. 2012;27:2160–8.
22. Smith GD, Silva E, Silva CA. Developmental consequences of cryopreservation of mammalian oocytes and embryos. Reprod Biomed Online. 2004;9(2):171–8.
23. Ebner T, Moser M, Sommergruber M, Gaiswinkler U, Shebl O, Jesacher K, Tews G. Occurrence and developmental consequences of vacuoles throughout preimplantation development. Fertil Steril. 2005;83(6):1635–40.
24. Hyttel P, Vajta G, Callesen H. Vitrification of bovine oocytes with the open pulled straw method: ultrastructural consequences. Mol Reprod Dev. 2000;56(1):80–8.
25. Wu C, Rui R, Dai J, Zhang C, Ju S, Xie B, Lu X, Zheng X. Effects of cryopreservation on the developmental competence, ultrastructure and cytoskeletal structure of porcine oocytes. Mol Reprod Dev. 2006;73(11):1454–62.
26. Boonkusol D, Faisaikarm T, Dinnyes A, Kitiyanant Y. Effects of vitrification procedures on subsequent development and ultrastructure of in-vitro matured swamp buffalo (Bubalus bubalis) oocytes. Reprod Fertil Dev. 2007;19(2):383–91.
27. Paynter SJ, O'Neil L, Fuller BJ, Shaw RW. Membrane permeability of human oocytes in the presence of the cryoprotectant propane-1,2-diol. Fertil Steril. 2001;75(3):532–8.

28. Kleinhans FW. Membrane permeability modelling: Kedem-Katchalsky vs a two-parameter formalism. Cryobiology. 1998;37(4):271–89.
29. Leibo SP. Water permeability and its activation energy of fertilized and unfertilized mouse ova. J Membr Biol. 1980;53(3):179–88.
30. Newton H, Pegg DE, Barrass R, Gosden RG. Osmotically inactive volume, hydraulic conductivity, and permeability to dimethyl sulfoxide of human mature oocytes. J Reprod Fertil. 1999;117(1):27–33.
31. Mazur P. Kinetics of water loss from cells at subzero temperatures and the likelihood of intracellular freezing. J Gen Physiol. 1963;47:347–69.
32. Fuller B, Paynter S. Fundamentals of cryobiology in reproductive medicine. Reprod Biomed Online. 2004;9:680–91.
33. Arav A. Cryopreservation of oocytes and embryos. Theriogenology. 2014;81(1):96–102.
34. Vajta G, Nagy ZP. Are programmable freezers still needed in the embryo laboratory? Review on vitrification. Reprod Biomed Online. 2006;12:779–96.
35. Vajta G. Vitrification in human and domestic animal embryology: work in progress. Reprod Fertil Dev. 2013;25:719–27.
36. Vajta G, Reichart A, Ubaldi F, Rienzi L. From a backup technology to a strategy-outlining approach: the success story of cryopreservation 2013. Expert Rev Obst Gynecol. 2013;8:181–90.
37. Mori C, Yabuuchi A, Ezoe K, Murata N, Takayama Y, Okimura T, Uchiyama K, Takakura K, Abe H, Wada K, Okuno T, Kobayashi T, Kato K. Hydroxypropyl cellulose as an option for supplementation of cryoprotectant solutions for embryo vitrification in human assisted reproductive technologies. Reprod Biomed Online. 2015;30:613–21.
38. Papis K, Shimizu M, Izaike Y. Factors affecting the survivability of bovine oocytes vitrified in droplets. Theriogenology. 2000;54:651–8.
39. Vajta G, Holm P, Kuwayama M, Booth PJ, Jacobsen H, Greve T, Callesen H. Open Pulled Straw (OPS) vitrification: a new way to reduce cryoinjuries of bovine ova and embryos. Mol Reprod Dev. 1998;51:53–8.
40. Seki S, Mazur P. Effect of warming rate on the survival of vitrified mouse oocytes and on the recrystallization of intracellular ice. Biol Reprod. 2008;79:727–37.
41. Seki S, Mazur P. The dominance of warming rate over cooling rate in the survival of mouse oocytes subjected to a vitrification procedure. Cryobiology. 2009;59:75–82.
42. Mazur P, Seki S. Survival of mouse oocytes after being cooled in a vitrification solution to −196 degrees C at 95 degrees to 70,000 degrees C/min and warmed at 610 degrees to 118,000 degrees C/min: a new paradigm for cryopreservation by vitrification. Cryobiology. 2011;62:1–7.
43. Stoop D, De MN, Jansen E, Platteau P, Van den Abbeel E, Verheyen G, Devroey P. Clinical validation of a closed vitrification system in an oocyte-donation programme. Reprod Biomed Online. 2012;24:180–5.
44. Papatheodorou A, Vanderzwalmen P, Panagiotidis Y, Prapas N, Zikopoulos K, Georgiou I, Prapas Y. Open versus closed oocyte vitrification system: a prospective randomized sibling oocyte study. Reprod Biomed Online. 2013;26:595–602.
45. Panagiotidis Y, Vanderzwalmen P, Prapas Y, Kasapi E, Goudakou M, Papatheodorou A, Passadaki T, Petousis S, Nikolettos N, Veletza S, Prapas N, Maroulis G. Open versus closed vitrification of blastocysts from an oocyte-donation programme: a prospective randomized study. Reprod Biomed Online. 2013;26:470–6.
46. Yavin S, Arav A. Measurement of essential physical properties of vitrification solutions. Theriogenology. 2007;67:81–9.
47. Martino A, Songsasen N, Leibo SP. Development into blastocysts of bovine oocytes cryopreserved by ultra-rapid cooling. Biol Reprod. 1996;54:1059–69.
48. Bielanski A, Vajta G. Risk of contamination of germplasm during cryopreservation and cryobanking in IVF units. Hum Reprod. 2009;24:2457–67.

49. Vajta G, Rienzi L, Ubaldi FM. Open versus closed systems for vitrification of human oocytes and embryos. Reprod Biomed Online. 2015;30:325–33.
50. Vajta G, Lewis IM, Kuwayama M, Greve T, Callesen H. Sterile application of the Open Pulled Straw (OPS) vitrification method. Cryo Letters. 1998;19:389–92.
51. Cobo A, Romero JL, Perez S, de los Santos MJ, Meseguer M, Remohi J. Storage of human oocytes in the vapor phase of nitrogen. Fertil Steril. 2010;94:1903–7.
52. Parmegiani L, Accorsi A, Bernardi S, Arnone A, Cognigni GE, Filicori M. A reliable procedure for decontamination before thawing of human specimens cryostored in liquid nitrogen: three washes with sterile liquid nitrogen (SLN(2)). Fertil Steril. 2012;98:870–5.

Chapter 9
Optimal Preparation Prior to the Use of Cryopreserved Oocytes

Shari Mackens, Arne van de Vijver, and Samuel Santos-Ribeiro

The early 1980s saw the first cases of live births after the transfer of autologous frozen embryos be reported [1, 2]. These preliminary reports were met with reasonable resistance by the scientific community owing to the limited efficacy of earlier cryopreservation methods and concerns regarding the overall safety of embryo cryopreservation. This uncertainty effectively relayed embryo cryopreservation at its genesis to the status of an "adjuvant method" for cycles in which the number of embryos produced was deemed too excessive for simultaneous replacement during the fresh embryo transfer (ET) attempt. However, following the advent of more efficient cryopreservation strategies [3] (*i.e.* vitrification) and reassuring safety data [4, 5], the use of embryo cryopreservation has progressively increased, currently accounting for up to one third of all children born after assisted reproductive technologies (ART) in the United States [6]. Furthermore, cryopreservation has now become an indispensable tool in everyday clinical practice, providing the necessary means to assure the safe storage of embryos while minimizing the many risks associated to the multiple pregnancies [7]. For this reason, an increasing amount of scientific societies and governments have encouraged [8] or even enforced [9, 10] elective single ET policies to ART clinics, progressively changing

S. Mackens, M.D. (✉) • A. van de Vijver, M.D., PhD
Centre for Reproductive Medicine, Universitair Ziekenhuis Brussel, Vrije Universiteit Brussel, Brussels 1090, Belgium
e-mail: Shari.Mackens@uzbrussel.be

S. Santos-Ribeiro, M.D.
Centre for Reproductive Medicine, Universitair Ziekenhuis Brussel, Vrije Universiteit Brussel, Brussels 1090, Belgium

Department of Obstetrics, Gynaecology and Reproductive Medicine, Santa Maria University Hospital, Lisbon 1649-035, Portugal

© Springer International Publishing Switzerland 2018
D. Stoop (ed.), *Preventing Age Related Fertility Loss*,
DOI 10.1007/978-3-319-14857-1_9

the benchmark of ART from *pregnancy rates* to *Birth Emphasizing a Successful Singleton at Term* (BESST) [11]. These considerations have set the stage for a new stance on embryo cryopreservation in modern-day medicine, which is no longer viewed as a simple adjuvant of fresh ET [12], a mindset that has transpired across to oocyte donation and/or embryo cryopreservation programs as well. In parallel, an increasing number of women are currently opting to electively cryopreserve oocytes in anticipation of age-related gamete exhaustion. Since the first live birth following the transfer of a cryopreserved oocyte occurred already in 1986 [13], physicians have the possibility to extrapolate from the abundance of data already existent from both fresh/frozen oocyte donation and embryo cryopreservation programs in order to determine the best ET strategy for women thawing electively cryopreserved oocytes. In this chapter, we give a detailed explanation on how the preparation of the uterus for the transfer of embryos deriving from cryopreserved oocytes is generally performed, followed by a brief overview of which methods one may consider to optimize the safety and pregnancy/neonatal outcomes of these treatment cycles.

Types of Embryo Transfer Protocols

The transfer of an embryo deriving from cryopreserved oocytes poses several potential advantages, the most important of which is the fact that the attention of the physician is no longer divided between both the maximization of oocyte retrieval and the optimization of uterine receptivity. This allows physicians to opt for more patient-friendly alternatives of endometrial preparation which frequently no longer involve the daily administration of injectable drugs. Instead, doctors usually choose to use either oral or intravaginal hormone therapy (artificial cycle) or even to simply monitor the menstrual cycle to determine the best timing for the thawing and transfer without medication (natural cycle).

Artificial Cycle

Artificial hormonal therapy cycles are frequently used for endometrium preparation for an ET. This treatment protocol, which was originally developed for patients undergoing oocyte donation, has also proven to be successful in the general population of women undergoing ETs [14]. Taking into account the minimal cycle monitoring related to such a practice (*i.e.* hormonal analyses and ultrasound scans of the endometrium), exogenous estrogen and progesterone administration for ET preparation has become increasingly popular. On the other hand, potential disadvantages associated to this approach include the cost, inconvenience, prolonged treatment (especially in case of pregnancy) and potential side-effects associated to estrogen supplementation (*e.g.* increased thrombotic risk).

Estrogen Supplementation

The scarce evidence available on this topic has shown that even a relatively short period of estrogen supplementation of 5–7 days seems to be sufficient for adequate endometrial proliferation [15]. However, most artificial cycle protocols still empirically opt to extend the duration of estrogen supplementation to approximately 2 weeks to better mimic the natural menstrual cycle. Furthermore, if necessary (*e.g.* due to a persistently thin endometrium), the duration of estrogen supplementation can be prolonged until up to 7 weeks without compromising ET pregnancy outcome [16].

Progesterone Supplementation

Once the proliferation of the endometrium with the administration of estrogen is considered adequate (*i.e.* when the endometrial thickness on ultrasound is around 6–7 mm), progesterone is initiated to promote the final phase of endometrial preparation prior to embryo transfer. The optimal duration of exposure to progesterone prior to ET is, however, currently also an elusive topic [17], namely in oocyte donation programs [18]. In a natural cycle, progesterone rises to 1–3 ng/mL 2–3 days before ovulation, due to the LH-stimulated production by the peripheral granulosa cells [19], with a steep increase in production following ovulation (3–10 ng/mL). However, the clinical importance of this pre-ovulatory progesterone elevation is yet to be determined. Furthermore, when progesterone supplementation in artificial cycles is initiated 3 days before the ET [20, 21], excellent pregnancy rates of up to 40.5% still occur [22]. Indeed, some evidence demonstrating pregnancies after very short durations of progesterone supplementation indicate that short progesterone exposure may suffice to induce endometrial receptivity [23, 24]. On the order hand, a recent randomized controlled trial (RCT) revealed that transferring day-4 embryos on the third day of progesterone supplementation was deleterious [25]. Specifically, a higher risk of early pregnancy loss was seen during the study, possibly caused either by the asynchrony between the duration of progesterone administration and the developmental stage of the embryo or by an insufficient endometrial decidualization associated with only 3 days of progesterone administration (which could potentially still allow implantation to occur but then increase early pregnancy loss). Finally, a recent study highlighted once again the importance of optimal progesterone exposure timing by showing an increase in pregnancy rates associated with specific histological endometrial dating patterns and corresponding adjustments in progesterone exposure [26]. Currently, most of the cleavage stage embryos are empirically transferred around the fourth day of progesterone supplementation, whereas blastocysts are usually transferred on the sixth day of progesterone supplementation. Practically, this means that vitrified oocytes are warmed on the second or first day of the progesterone supplementation [27, 28]. The clinical outcome of these different durations of progesterone supplementation before transfer was not significantly different in fresh oocyte donation cycles, however, a higher rate of biochemical pregnancies was seen when supplementing progesterone 1 day before oocyte retrieval [18]. More evidence is needed to confirm best clinical practice.

In most clinics progesterone supplementation is routinely administered vaginally by micronized progesterone (200 mg three times daily) with the most frequent side effect being vaginal irritation and discharge. Non-inferiority and a similar safety profile have been recently demonstrated for the oral administration of dydrogesterone (10 mg three times daily) [29], although concern was raised in the past because of a positive association between dydrogesterone usage during early pregnancy and congenital heart disease in the offspring [30].

Natural Cycle

In regular-cycling women, an alternative to artificial cycles may be to monitor the menstrual cycle and schedule the transfer for the moment when the endometrium is "synchronized" to the developmental stage of the embryo. The starting point to assess embryo-endometrial synchronization is normally the ovulation of the dominant follicle, which in an ET cycle can either be triggered exogenously (*i.e.* modified natural cycles, in which ovulation is triggered by the administration of human chorionic gonadotropin (hCG) as soon as a dominant follicle of *e.g.* >16 mm is observed on ultrasound monitoring) or by serial blood (or, albeit less accurately, urine) sampling until a LH peak is observed [31]. In accordance with the planning of ET in an artificial cycle [27, 28], oocytes are warmed 3 or 2 days after the LH peak/hCG trigger in a natural cycle.

When pitting natural cycles against artificial cycles, one is opting between (a) the transfer of an embryo into an endometrium altered the least possible by external factors and (b) a less cumbersome approach that requires less clinic visits and allows for more flexibility in terms of cycle scheduling. In terms of pregnancy rates, a recent RCT including 1032 women and comparing artificial and modified natural cycles failed to show any significant difference between both approaches [32]. At first glance, this study seems to indicate that the choice in terms of the type of ET to perform could be based exclusively on patient/physician choice; however, this study did not assess the potential benefit of ETs performed without exogenous ovulation triggering. On this matter, two small RCT revealed conflicting results: the first (which included 60 cycles) did not find significant differences between spontaneous and exogenously-triggered ovulation cycles [33], while the other (planned to include 240 women) was interrupted prematurely (after recruiting 124 women) due to the fact that an interim analysis revealed a remarkably lower pregnancy rates in women who were administered hCG for ovulation (14.3% vs. 31.4%, respectively) [31]. One of the posited reasons for this difference was the fact that the researchers had considered different timings to perform the ET (specifically, a 1-day difference between both studies); however, a recent large retrospective analysis also associated LH peak ovulation ET cycles with better pregnancy outcomes even when using a comparable transfer schedule Scheme [34]. That said, until further prospective studies comparing non-modified natural cycles with artificial cycles are performed, a final decision on what seems the best type of ET remains unanswered.

Embryo Transfer Outcome Optimization

Human embryo implantation is currently the rate-limiting step of ART. The transferred embryo and the maternal endometrium are the two key-players and a synchronous interaction between a competent embryo and a receptive endometrium is indispensable for successful implantation. In the natural menstrual cycle, the endometrial window of implantation *opens* 6 days after the postovulatory progesterone surge and lasts approximately 2–4 days [35]. During this window, the stepwise process of embryo implantation occurs. Specifically, first there is an apposition and adherence of the blastocyst to the endometrium, followed by the breaching of the luminal epithelium. Finally, the blastocyst invades the maternal tissue [36].

Ideally, when preparing the endometrium for ET, one would be able to assess if it is receptive (*i.e.* if it is in the window of implantation). Unfortunately, despite enormous research in the field, a test for endometrial receptivity at the molecular level is still not widely accessible or validated at this time. Therefore, ultrasonography and endocrine monitoring, being non-invasive and universally available, currently serve as surrogate markers to evaluate the endometrial status prior to transfer.

The endometrium requires adequate growth to allow successful implantation. A lower probability of pregnancy has been described for women with a thin endometrium [37], although this remains a topic of discussion [38]. Furthermore, a trilaminar endometrium on the day corresponding to the ovulation trigger day is associated with an increased probability of pregnancy [39].

Although the exact mechanism is unclear, a thin endometrium may be caused by the impairment of normal endometrial growth [40]. A number of treatments (including hysteroscopic adhesiolysis, hormonal manipulation by estrogen and GnRH-agonist, vasoactive drug such as aspirin, vitamin E, pentoxifylline, l-arginine or sildenafil, intra-uterine infusions of growth factors such as G-CSF and the application of regenerative medicine) have been proposed to stimulate endometrial growth in patients with a thin endometrium, but without much success [40, 41].

In addition to the thin endometrium, other women with no apparent problem in terms of endometrial growth and development still fail to reach implantation after multiple transfers of good quality embryos. Specifically, these women may suffer from repeated implantation failure (RIF), defined as the absence of implantation after two consecutive cycles of IVF, ICSI or frozen ET cycles in which the cumulative number of embryos previously transferred embryo was no less than four cleavage-stage embryos or two blastocysts (all of which should have been of good quality and appropriate developmental stage) [42]. Evidence-based diagnostic and therapeutic interventions for this group of patients remain even more limited, as the underlying reasons for implantation failure are largely unknown.

Ovarian Stimulation

Exogenous ovarian stimulation has been given to women undergoing ETs in an attempt to increase the circulation of serum estrogen and potentially enhance endometrial receptivity. However, a recent systematic review pooling the relevant data concluded that, when compared to unstimulated natural ET cycles, ovarian stimulation with gonadotropins or clomiphene citrate did not seem to enhance live birth pregnancy rates [43]. Interestingly, when compared to artificial cycles, women who performed ovarian stimulation with gonadotropins or letrozole did seem to have a slightly increased chance for live birth. However, until well-designed prospective studies are performed, no definitive recommendation on the use of ovarian stimulation in ET cycles can be made.

GnRH Agonist Downregulation

Besides the administration of estrogen and progesterone, a GnRH agonist is often added to the artificial cycle protocol, in order to prevent spontaneous ovulation. In a RCT encompassing 234 patients, cycles without ovarian suppression using a GnRH agonist were associated with a reduced clinical pregnancy and live birth rates per cycle [44], mainly due to a higher cycle cancellation rate. However, endocrine cycle monitoring was not performed in that study, and data with regard to the incidence of premature ovulation were not available. Furthermore, the results of this trial are strongly in contradiction with those of a subsequent systematic review and meta-analysis, which included an additional 491 patients deriving from another 3 RCT, could not demonstrate any benefit in terms of clinical pregnancy and cancellation rates [45]. Indeed, all three of these other RCT included in the meta-analysis failed to find any significant difference in terms of clinical pregnancy rates [46–48] among those in which the GnRH agonist was not administered. Similarly, another systematic review evaluating clinical pregnancy rates in women undergoing ET with frozen embryos or embryos derived from donor oocytes had similar results, failing again to reveal any significant benefit in using downregulation [49]. Finally, a more recent retrospective analysis of 1129 ET cycles also could not show any difference in live birth rates in cycles with or without GnRH agonist downregulation [50]. Adding to the overwhelming before-mentioned evidence, ET cycles without GnRH agonist co-treatment seem also to be more patient-friendly because of the avoidance of the cost and potential side effects associated with these drugs such as hot flashes, fatigue and other symptoms of estrogen deprivation.

Implantation Promoting Medications

Low Molecular Weight Heparins (LMWH) are thought to enhance endometrial receptivity by activating growth factors and cytokines that favor implantation. However, the clinical benefit of using LMWH in the peri-implantation period to increase pregnancy and live-birth rates is unclear. Importantly, since most studies inadequately reported adverse events, the safety of this strategy remains in question [51].

The use of corticosteroid therapy has also been attempted in ART, with the rationale that this immunosuppressant drug group could promote implantation (and reduce miscarriage) stemming from an oversimplification of the theory that an immune tolerance must be induced towards the invading embryo. However, the more this role of the immune system in implantation is unraveled, the more it becomes clear that a certain grade of inflammation and activation is actually required during the process. For this reason, immunologists are increasingly advocating that immune suppression should be reserved to women with overt immune pathology, especially given the fact that, besides the unproven benefit, these drugs may alter fetal growth and increase the risk of congenital anomalies and preterm birth [52, 53].

Endometrial Scratching and Hysteroscopy

The rationale for *endometrial scratching* first derived from observations in mice showing higher implantation rates following an intentional endometrial injury performed in the weeks preceding the window of implantation [54]. The molecular mechanism behind how the scratching of the endometrium could improve implantation is unclear at this time, although several hypotheses have thus far been advanced (*e.g.* resynchronizing of the endometrium, modulating the endometrial immune system) [55].

A systematic review published in 2015 compiling the relevant human clinical data until then concluded that endometrial scratching might result in better clinical pregnancy and live-birth rates in women with more than two previous failed ETs [56]. However, the interpretation of this data may be prone to bias due to the many differences in the trials that were included in the analysis (namely in terms of the timing, method and frequency of the endometrial scratching procedure that was performed), thus creating the need for further well-designed studies in these specific groups of patients.

Importantly, the only prospective study evaluating the effect of endometrial scratching during the transfer of an embryo in an unstimulated cycle (in which the procedure was performed in the preceding luteal phase) did not show any benefit in terms of implantation or clinical pregnancy rates [57].

Instead of routine endometrial scratching (which is generally performed by means of a blind endometrial biopsy), some researchers have attempted to focus on the effect of hysteroscopy to improve implantation in IVF. Nonetheless, the two largest and most recent trials did not show once again any significant effect in both women with RIF [58] or an unselected population [59].

Molecular Diagnostics

Approximately 15 years ago, researchers began to use high-throughput transcriptional data derived from endometrial biopsies to learn more about implantation in human reproduction. Currently, although many studies have been published on the subject, the use of this molecular diagnostic tool in clinical practice remains limited.

The endometrial receptivity array (ERA) is a molecular tool developed by Igenomix® (Valencia, Spain) to evaluate endometrial receptivity. This array analyses the expression of 238 genes on an endometrial biopsy [60] and, according to its expression pattern, a specifically designed predictor classifies the endometrium as 'receptive', 'pre-receptive' or 'post-receptive' [61]. The result of the analysis is thus an attempt to determine whether or not the patient is responsive to embryo implantation at the timing of sampling.

The endometrial tissue biopsy can be performed in either a natural or artificial cycle. The endometrial preparation is done just as it would be for an ET, but instead of an ET, an endometrial biopsy is performed.

In case of a receptive result, the transfer of a blastocyst should be performed in a subsequent ET cycle on the same day in which the biopsy was retrieved. For a day-3 embryo, the transfer should be anticipated by 2 days. Otherwise, if the ERA reveals that the endometrium was non-receptive at the time of biopsy, the expression profile can still be used to indicate on which day a second biopsy should be performed in order to validate the displacement of the window of implantation.

In women with RIF, a higher prevalence of the pre-receptive profile is generally suspected [62, 63]. Hence, when a displaced window of implantation is confirmed, implantation rates could potentially be increased by personalizing the day of the ET.

To strengthen the value of the ERA test and to validate its clinical applicability, the developing research group has currently two ongoing trials. A first (NCT01668693) started in 2012 and was designed to evaluate the efficacy of ERA and personalized ET in RIF patients. A second one (NCT01954758), initiated in 2013, is assessing the clinical value of ERA and personalized ET in a general population seeking IVF/ICSI treatment.

Very recently, another molecular signature consisting of 303 genes was developed to identify RIF patients [64]. The set of genes suggest that RIF is associated with reduced cell proliferation. The profile seems to stratify RIF patients into distinct groups with different subsequent implantation success rates. The analysis of the gene signature is currently not commercially available, but might also become of clinical value in the future.

Safety Concerns

Oocyte donation has been associated with a higher risk of adverse obstetric and neonatal outcomes, namely preeclampsia, low birth weight and preterm birth [65]. Having said that, one can question whether performing a ET using frozen oocytes/embryos (instead of a fresh transfer) impacts these risks further and in which manner?

Low birth weight (LBW) and preterm birth (PTB) are more prevalent following IVF/ICSI than after natural conception, even when only singleton pregnancies are taken into account [66]. Studies evaluating the transfer of frozen embryos, however, have shown that this strategy may significantly reduce the incidence of both [67, 68]. The explanation of this finding is not completely clear; however, experiments in mice have shown an altered fetal and placental development after ovarian stimulation for IVF [69–71]. This effect may not be of the same importance in oocyte donation cycles, since no ovarian stimulation is generally ever administered to the recipient [72]. On the other hand, besides the effect of the ovarian stimulation, one must also take into account that oocyte/embryo vitrification by itself serves indirectly as an selection method, possibly leading to better embryo quality and therefore better obstetrical outcome.

No difference between fresh and frozen transfer was found for stillbirth or perinatal mortality; however, a higher caesarian section rate was observed for frozen ET [67, 73]. Possible reasons for this may be that women undergoing frozen ET were more likely to have had a previous cesarean section compared with women undergoing fresh ET. Alternatively, following multiple failed IVF/ICSI attempts, these women may also be more likely to have cesarean sections performed given the false sense of higher safety frequently associated to this route of delivery [67].

The risk for major congenital anomalies is reported to be the same in children after fresh or frozen ET [74]. Furthermore, recent data showed that vitrification also does not seem to adversely affect the neonatal health of the offspring in comparison with transfer of fresh embryos. Specifically, in a recent retrospective analysis, neonatal health parameters (including the prevalence of congenital malformations) in singletons and twins born after embryo vitrification were similar or slightly better than those after fresh ET [4].

In the specific subgroup of polycystic ovary syndrome patients, a higher livebirth rate, mediated through a lower rate of pregnancy loss, was detected after frozen ET compared to fresh transfer. However, a higher risk of preeclampsia was also observed [75]. This is in line with the higher risk for pregnancy-induced hypertension observed in other studies [76–78]. However, the clinical significance of these findings and the extrapolation to oocyte recipients requires further investigation.

Key Points

1. Oocyte cryopreservation using vitrification is an efficient, safe and indispensable tool in clinical practice attempting to overcome age-related fertility loss.
2. The transfer of an embryo derived from cryopreserved oocytes poses the advantage that oocyte retrieval and uterine receptivity do not need to be synchronized, allowing an optimal approach of both.
3. Endometrial preparation prior the transfer of an embryo derived from cryopreserved oocytes can be done in a more patient-friendly fashion (without the daily administration of injectable drugs), by either oral or intravaginal hormone therapy (artificial cycle) or by simply monitoring the menstrual cycle to determine the best timing for the thawing and transfer without medication (natural cycle).
4. Further optimization to achieve higher success rates after embryo transfer (*e.g.* ovarian stimulation, GnRH agonist downregulation, implantation promoting medications, scratching/hysteroscopy) are often not evidence based and still under research. The same goes, at this time, for molecular diagnostic tools.

5. Oocyte donation is associated with a higher risk of adverse obstetric and neonatal outcomes, but performing an ET using frozen oocytes/embryos (instead of a fresh transfer) does not clearly impact these risks any further.

References

1. Trounson A, Mohr L. Human pregnancy following cryopreservation, thawing and transfer of an eight-cell embryo. Nature. 1983;305(5936):707–9.
2. Zeilmaker GH, Alberda AT, van Gent I, Rijkmans CM, Drogendijk AC. Two pregnancies following transfer of intact frozen-thawed embryos. Fertil Steril. 1984;42(2):293–6.
3. Balaban B, Urman B, Ata B, Isiklar A, Larman MG, Hamilton R, et al. A randomized controlled study of human Day 3 embryo cryopreservation by slow freezing or vitrification: vitrification is associated with higher survival, metabolism and blastocyst formation. Hum Reprod. 2008;23(9):1976–82.
4. Belva F, Bonduelle M, Roelants M, Verheyen G, Van Landuyt L. Neonatal health including congenital malformation risk of 1072 children born after vitrified embryo transfer. Hum Reprod. 2016;31(7):1610–20.
5. Belva F, Henriet S, Van den Abbeel E, Camus M, Devroey P, Van der Elst J, et al. Neonatal outcome of 937 children born after transfer of cryopreserved embryos obtained by ICSI and IVF and comparison with outcome data of fresh ICSI and IVF cycles. Hum Reprod. 2008;23(10):2227–38.
6. Doody KJ. Cryopreservation and delayed embryo transfer-assisted reproductive technology registry and reporting implications. Fertil Steril. 2014;102(1):27–31.
7. Pandian Z, Marjoribanks J, Ozturk O, Serour G, Bhattacharya S. Number of embryos for transfer following in vitro fertilisation or intra-cytoplasmic sperm injection. Cochrane Database Syst Rev. 2013;7:CD003416.
8. Maheshwari A, Griffiths S, Bhattacharya S. Global variations in the uptake of single embryo transfer. Hum Reprod Update. 2011;17(1):107–20.
9. Peeraer K, Debrock S, Laenen A, De Loecker P, Spiessens C, De Neubourg D, et al. The impact of legally restricted embryo transfer and reimbursement policy on cumulative delivery rate after treatment with assisted reproduction technology. Hum Reprod. 2014;29(2):267–75.
10. Sundstrom P, Saldeen P. Cumulative delivery rate in an in vitro fertilization program with a single embryo transfer policy. Acta Obstet Gynecol Scand. 2009;88(6):700–6.
11. Min JK. What is the most relevant standard of success in assisted reproduction? The singleton, term gestation, live birth rate per cycle initiated: the BESST endpoint for assisted reproduction. Hum Reprod. 2004;19(1):3–7.
12. Blockeel C, Drakopoulos P, Santos-Ribeiro S, Polyzos NP, Tournaye H. A fresh look at the freeze-all protocol: a SWOT analysis. Hum Reprod. 2016;31(3):491–7.
13. Chen C. Pregnancy after human oocyte cryopreservation. Lancet. 1986;1(8486):884–6.
14. Younis JS, Simon A, Laufer N. Endometrial preparation: lessons from oocyte donation. Fertil Steril. 1996;66(6):873–84.
15. Navot D, Laufer N, Kopolovic J, Rabinowitz R, Birkenfeld A, Lewin A, et al. Artificially induced endometrial cycles and establishment of pregnancies in the absence of ovaries. N Engl J Med. 1986;314(13):806–11.
16. Soares SR, Troncoso C, Bosch E, Serra V, Simon C, Remohi J, et al. Age and uterine receptiveness: predicting the outcome of oocyte donation cycles. J Clin Endocrinol Metab. 2005;90(7):4399–404.
17. Nawroth F, Ludwig M. What is the 'ideal' duration of progesterone supplementation before the transfer of cryopreserved-thawed embryos in estrogen/progesterone replacement protocols? Hum Reprod. 2005;20(5):1127–34.

18. Escriba MJ, Bellver J, Bosch E, Sanchez M, Pellicer A, Remohi J. Delaying the initiation of progesterone supplementation until the day of fertilization does not compromise cycle outcome in patients receiving donated oocytes: a randomized study. Fertil Steril. 2006;86(1):92–7.
19. Fritz MA, Speroff L. Regulation of the menstrual cycle. In: Fritz MA, Speroff L, editors. Clinical gynecologic endocrinology and infertility. 8th ed. Philadelphia: Lippincott Williams and Wilkins; 2011. p. 199–242.
20. Boldt J, Cline D, McLaughlin D. Human oocyte cryopreservation as an adjunct to IVF-embryo transfer cycles. Hum Reprod. 2003;18(6):1250–5.
21. Revel A, Safran A, Laufer N, Lewin A, Reubinov BE, Simon A. Twin delivery following 12 years of human embryo cryopreservation: case report. Hum Reprod. 2004;19(2):328–9.
22. Givens CR, Markun LC, Ryan IP, Chenette PE, Herbert CM, Schriock ED. Outcomes of natural cycles versus programmed cycles for 1677 frozen-thawed embryo transfers. Reprod Biomed Online. 2009;19(3):380–4.
23. Imbar T, Hurwitz A. Synchronization between endometrial and embryonic age is not absolutely crucial for implantation. Fertil Steril. 2004;82(2):472–4.
24. Theodorou E, Forman R. Live birth after blastocyst transfer following only 2 days of progesterone administration in an agonadal oocyte recipient. Reprod Biomed Online. 2012;25(4):355–7.
25. van de Vijver A, Polyzos NP, Van Landuyt L, Mackens S, Stoop D, Camus M, et al. What is the optimal duration of progesterone administration before transferring a vitrified-warmed cleavage stage embryo? A randomized controlled trial. Hum Reprod. 2016;31(5):1097–104.
26. Gomaa H, Casper RF, Esfandiari N, Bentov Y. Non-synchronized endometrium and its correction in non-ovulatory cryopreserved embryo transfer cycles. Reprod Biomed Online. 2015;30(4):378–84.
27. Stoop D, De Munck N, Jansen E, Platteau P, Van den Abbeel E, Verheyen G, Devroey P. Clinical validation of a closed vitrification system in an oocyte-donation programme. Reprod Biomed Online. 2012;24(2):180–5.
28. Cobo A, Meseguer M, Remohi J, Pellicer A. Use of cryo-banked oocytes in an ovum donation programme: a prospective, randomized, controlled, clinical trial. Hum Reprod. 2010;25(9):2239–46.
29. Tournaye H, Gennady TS, Kahler E, Griesinger G. A Phase III randomized controlled trial comparing the efficacy, safety and tolerability of oral dydrogesterone versus micronized vaginal progesterone for luteal support in in vitro fertilization. Hum Reprod. 2017;32(5):1019–27.
30. Zaqout M, Aslem E, Abuqamar M, Abughazza O, Panzer J, De Wolf D. The impact of oral intake of dydrogesterone on fetal heart development during early pregnancy. Pediatr Cardiol. 2015;36(7):1483–8.
31. Fatemi HM, Kyrou D, Bourgain C, Van den Abbeel E, Griesinger G, Devroey P. Cryopreserved-thawed human embryo transfer: spontaneous natural cycle is superior to human chorionic gonadotropin-induced natural cycle. Fertil Steril. 2010;94(6):2054–8.
32. Groenewoud ER, Cohlen BJ, Al-Oraiby A, Brinkhuis EA, Broekmans FJ, de Bruin JP, et al. A randomized controlled, non-inferiority trial of modified natural versus artificial cycle for cryo-thawed embryo transfer. Hum Reprod. 2016;31(7):1483–92.
33. Weissman A, Horowitz E, Ravhon A, Steinfeld Z, Mutzafi R, Golan A, et al. Spontaneous ovulation versus HCG triggering for timing natural-cycle frozen-thawed embryo transfer: a randomized study. Reprod Biomed Online. 2011;23(4):484–9.
34. Montagut M, Santos-Ribeiro S, De Vos M, Polyzos NP, Drakopoulos P, Mackens S, et al. Frozen-thawed embryo transfers in natural cycles with spontaneous or induced ovulation: the search for the best protocol continues. Hum Reprod. 2016;31(12):2803–10.
35. Teklenburg G, Salker M, Molokhia M, Lavery S, Trew G, Aojanepong T, et al. Natural selection of human embryos: decidualizing endometrial stromal cells serve as sensors of embryo quality upon implantation. PLoS One. 2010;5(4):e10258.
36. Quenby S, Brosens JJ. Human implantation: a tale of mutual maternal and fetal attraction. Biol Reprod. 2013;88(3):81.

37. Mahajan N, Sharma S. The endometrium in assisted reproductive technology: how thin is thin? J Human Reprod Sci. 2016;9(1):3–8.
38. Dain L, Bider D, Levron J, Zinchenko V, Westler S, Dirnfeld M. Thin endometrium in donor oocyte recipients: enigma or obstacle for implantation? Fertil Steril. 2013;100(5):1289–95.
39. Grunfeld L, Walker B, Bergh PA, Sandler B, Hofmann G, Navot D. High-resolution endovaginal ultrasonography of the endometrium: a noninvasive test for endometrial adequacy. Obstet Gynecol. 1991;78(2):200–4.
40. Miwa I, Tamura H, Takasaki A, Yamagata Y, Shimamura K, Sugino N. Pathophysiologic features of "thin" endometrium. Fertil Steril. 2009;91(4):998–1004.
41. Lebovitz O, Orvieto R. Treating patients with "thin" endometrium—an ongoing challenge. Gynecol Endocrinol. 2014;30(6):409–14.
42. Polanski LT, Baumgarten MN, Quenby S, Brosens J, Campbell BK, Raine-Fenning NJ. What exactly do we mean by 'recurrent implantation failure'? A systematic review and opinion. Reprod Biomed Online. 2014;28(4):409–23.
43. Yarali H, Polat M, Mumusoglu S, Yarali I, Bozdag G. Preparation of endometrium for frozen embryo replacement cycles: a systematic review and meta-analysis. J Assist Reprod Genet. 2016;33(10):1287–304.
44. El-Toukhy T, Taylor A, Khalaf Y, Al-Darazi K, Rowell P, Seed P, et al. Pituitary suppression in ultrasound-monitored frozen embryo replacement cycles. A randomised study. Hum Reprod. 2004;19(4):874–9.
45. Ghobara T, Vandekerckhove P. Cycle regimens for frozen-thawed embryo transfer. Cochrane Database Syst Rev. 2008;1:CD003414.
46. Dal Prato L, Borini A, Cattoli M, Bonu MA, Sciajno R, Flamigni C. Endometrial preparation for frozen-thawed embryo transfer with or without pretreatment with gonadotropin-releasing hormone agonist. Fertil Steril. 2002;77(5):956–60.
47. Loh SKE, Ganesan G, Leong N, editors. Clomid versus hormone endometrial preparation in FET cycles 17th World Congress on Fertility and Sterility (IFFS); 2001; Melbourne.
48. Simon A, Hurwitz A, Zentner BS, Bdolah Y, Laufer N. Transfer of frozen-thawed embryos in artificially prepared cycles with and without prior gonadotrophin-releasing hormone agonist suppression: a prospective randomized study. Hum Reprod. 1998;13(1O):2712–7.
49. Glujovsky D, Pesce R, Fiszbajn G, Sueldo C, Hart RJ, Ciapponi A. Endometrial preparation for women undergoing embryo transfer with frozen embryos or embryos derived from donor oocytes. Cochrane Database Syst Rev. 2010;1:CD006359.
50. van de Vijver A, Polyzos NP, Van Landuyt L, De Vos M, Camus M, Stoop D, et al. Cryopreserved embryo transfer in an artificial cycle: is GnRH agonist down-regulation necessary? Reprod Biomed Online. 2014;29(5):588–94.
51. Akhtar MA, Sur S, Raine-Fenning N, Jayaprakasan K, Thornton JG, Quenby S. Heparin for assisted reproduction. Cochrane Database Syst Rev. 2013;8:CD009452.
52. Moffett A, Shreeve N. First do no harm: uterine natural killer (NK) cells in assisted reproduction. Hum Reprod. 2015;30(7):1519–25.
53. Robertson SA, Jin M, Yu D, Moldenhauer LM, Davies MJ, Hull ML, et al. Corticosteroid therapy in assisted reproduction—immune suppression is a faulty premise. Hum Reprod. 2016;31(10):2164–73.
54. Zhang XH, Liu ZZ, Tang MX, Zhang YH, Hu L, Liao AH. Morphological changes and expression of cytokine after local endometrial injury in a mouse model. Reprod Sci. 2015;22(11):1377–86.
55. Gnainsky Y, Granot I, Aldo P, Barash A, Or Y, Mor G, et al. Biopsy-induced inflammatory conditions improve endometrial receptivity: the mechanism of action. Reproduction. 2015;149(1):75–85.
56. Nastri CO, Lensen SF, Gibreel A, Raine-Fenning N, Ferriani RA, Bhattacharya S, et al. Endometrial injury in women undergoing assisted reproductive techniques. Cochrane Database Syst Rev. 2015;3:CD009517.
57. Dunne C, Taylor B. Does endometrial injury improve implantation of frozen-thawed embryos? Arch Gynccol Obstet. 2014;290(3):575–9.

58. El-Toukhy T, Campo R, Khalaf Y, Tabanelli C, Gianaroli L, Gordts SS, et al. Hysteroscopy in recurrent in-vitro fertilisation failure (TROPHY): a multicentre, randomised controlled trial. Lancet. 2016;387(10038):2614–21.
59. Smit JG, Kasius JC, Eijkemans MJ, Koks CA, van Golde R, Nap AW, et al. Hysteroscopy before in-vitro fertilisation (inSIGHT): a multicentre, randomised controlled trial. Lancet. 2016;387(10038):2622–9.
60. Diaz-Gimeno P, Horcajadas JA, Martinez-Conejero JA, Esteban FJ, Alama P, Pellicer A, et al. A genomic diagnostic tool for human endometrial receptivity based on the transcriptomic signature. Fertil Steril. 2011;95(1):50–60.
61. Diaz-Gimeno P, Ruiz-Alonso M, Blesa D, Bosch N, Martinez-Conejero JA, Alama P, et al. The accuracy and reproducibility of the endometrial receptivity array is superior to histology as a diagnostic method for endometrial receptivity. Fertil Steril. 2013;99(2):508–17.
62. Ruiz-Alonso M, Blesa D, Diaz-Gimeno P, Gomez E, Fernandez-Sanchez M, Carranza F, et al. The endometrial receptivity array for diagnosis and personalized embryo transfer as a treatment for patients with repeated implantation failure. Fertil Steril. 2013;100(3):818–24.
63. Ruiz-Alonso M, Galindo N, Pellicer A, Simon C. What a difference two days make: "personalized" embryo transfer (pET) paradigm: a case report and pilot study. Hum Reprod. 2014;29(6):1244–7.
64. Koot YE, van Hooff SR, Boomsma CM, van Leenen D, Groot Koerkamp MJ, Goddijn M, et al. An endometrial gene expression signature accurately predicts recurrent implantation failure after IVF. Sci Rep. 2016;6:19411.
65. Storgaard M, Loft A, Bergh C, Wennerholm UB, Soderstrom-Anttila V, Romundstad LB, et al. Obstetric and neonatal complications in pregnancies conceived after oocyte donation—a systematic review and meta-analysis. BJOG. 2016;124(4):561–72.
66. Pinborg A, Wennerholm UB, Romundstad LB, Loft A, Aittomaki K, Soderstrom-Anttila V, et al. Why do singletons conceived after assisted reproduction technology have adverse perinatal outcome? Systematic review and meta-analysis. Hum Reprod Update. 2013;19(2):87–104.
67. Zhao J, Xu B, Zhang Q, Li YP. Which one has a better obstetric and perinatal outcome in singleton pregnancy, IVF/ICSI or FET?: a systematic review and meta-analysis. Reprod Biol Endocrinol. 2016;14(1):51.
68. Maheshwari A, Pandey S, Shetty A, Hamilton M, Bhattacharya S. Obstetric and perinatal outcomes in singleton pregnancies resulting from the transfer of frozen thawed versus fresh embryos generated through in vitro fertilization treatment: a systematic review and meta-analysis. Fertil Steril. 2012;98(2):368–77e1–9.
69. Bloise E, Lin W, Liu X, Simbulan R, Kolahi KS, Petraglia F, et al. Impaired placental nutrient transport in mice generated by in vitro fertilization. Endocrinology. 2012;153(7):3457–67.
70. Delle Piane L, Lin W, Liu X, Donjacour A, Minasi P, Revelli A, et al. Effect of the method of conception and embryo transfer procedure on mid-gestation placenta and fetal development in an IVF mouse model. Hum Reprod. 2010;25(8):2039–46.
71. Mainigi MA, Olalere D, Burd I, Sapienza C, Bartolomei M, Coutifaris C. Peri-implantation hormonal milieu: elucidating mechanisms of abnormal placentation and fetal growth. Biol Reprod. 2014;90(2):26.
72. Kalra SK, Ratcliffe SJ, Coutifaris C, Molinaro T, Barnhart KT. Ovarian stimulation and low birth weight in newborns conceived through in vitro fertilization. Obstet Gynecol. 2011;118(4):863–71.
73. Maheshwari A, Kalampokas T, Davidson J, Bhattacharya S. Obstetric and perinatal outcomes in singleton pregnancies resulting from the transfer of blastocyst-stage versus cleavage-stage embryos generated through in vitro fertilization treatment: a systematic review and meta-analysis. Fertil Steril. 2013;100(6):1615–21e1–10.
74. Pelkonen S, Hartikainen AL, Ritvanen A, Koivunen R, Martikainen H, Gissler M, et al. Major congenital anomalies in children born after frozen embryo transfer: a cohort study 1995–2006. Hum Reprod. 2014;29(7):1552–7.
75. Chen ZJ, Shi Y, Sun Y, Zhang B, Liang X, Cao Y, et al. Fresh versus frozen embryos for infertility in the polycystic ovary syndrome. N Engl J Med. 2016;375(6):523–33.

76. Opdahl S, Henningsen AA, Tiitinen A, Bergh C, Pinborg A, Romundstad PR, et al. Risk of hypertensive disorders in pregnancies following assisted reproductive technology: a cohort study from the CoNARTaS group. Hum Reprod. 2015;30(7):1724–31.
77. Sazonova A, Kallen K, Thurin-Kjellberg A, Wennerholm UB, Bergh C. Obstetric outcome in singletons after in vitro fertilization with cryopreserved/thawed embryos. Hum Reprod. 2012;27(5):1343–50.
78. Ishihara O, Araki R, Kuwahara A, Itakura A, Saito H, Adamson GD. Impact of frozen-thawed single-blastocyst transfer on maternal and neonatal outcome: an analysis of 277,042 single-embryo transfer cycles from 2008 to 2010 in Japan. Fertil Steril. 2014;101(1):128–33.

Chapter 10
Clinical Outcome After Oocyte Cryopreservation for Elective Fertility Preservation

Ana Cobo

Fertility preservation (FP) is an emerging, rapidly evolving branch of reproductive medicine comprising the preservation of gametes (sperm, oocytes), and reproductive tissue (ovarian, testicular), giving individuals at risk of losing their reproductive ability the chance to conceive and have their own genetic offspring. Cancer patients to undergo surgery or start chemotherapy or radiotherapy, other medical conditions leading to premature menopause, and healthy women wishing to postpone childbearing, are the main beneficiaries of this strategy. Options for women to safeguard their fertility include the cryopreservation of ovarian tissue or oocytes.

The preservation of biological materials at cryogenic temperatures (cryopreservation) allows complete stopping of biological reactions with the aim of preserving the viability of the cells while keeping intact the tissue physiology after the transplantation of organs or in the case of gametes, to preserve unaltered their ability to produce embryos able to generate viable pregnancies and healthy babies. Efficient cryopreservation of oocytes has helped greatly as a tool for FP especially during the last 10 years. More specifically, the introduction of vitrification into assisted reproduction (AR) has established efficient female gamete cryopreservation, which provides comparable outcomes to those achieved with fresh oocytes [1, 2] and opens up a wide range of applications, including FP [3].

Elective Fertility Preservation (EFP) for Social Reasons

In today's society, many women who are taking long strides in their careers and delaying pregnancy further away from the younger years of childbearing. This trend affects mainly the developed countries most of which are experiencing a

A. Cobo
IVI-Valencia, Institut Universitari IVI, Plaça de la Policia Local 3, Valencia, Spain
e-mail: ana.cobo@ivi.es

© Springer International Publishing Switzerland 2018

D. Stoop (ed.), *Preventing Age Related Fertility Loss*,
DOI 10.1007/978-3-319-14857-1_10

significantly reduced birth rate. Women are often forced to choose advancement of career, financial security, and certain social pressures ahead of their biological clock, the well-known decline in fertility over 30s. With more women deciding to delay motherhood, there is an increase interest in the availability of the current cryopreservation technologies in order to safeguard their options for the future.

A compilation of the first series of outcomes achieved when women who vitrified their oocytes due to EFP in our centres returned to attempt pregnancy was published in 2013, providing the first report on babies achieved after elective fertility preservation for social reasons [3]. Therefore, five babies were reported. Concomitantly, the birth of a baby boy whose mother had non-Hodgkin lymphoma when she vitrified her oocytes prior to the oncological treatment was also reported [3]. A more recent review of our data published in 2016 provide a detailed description of the situation of EFP in our group, including the profile of the woman who have vitrified, the rate at which they return to use their oocytes, their clinical outcomes and the probability of having a baby according to the number of oocytes consumed [4]. The study included 1468 women, while most of them (N = 1382) opted for EFP due to age related fertility decline (social reasons). The reason why the remaining women chose EFP (N = 86 patients) was the presence of a medical condition, other than cancer, which could undermine future fertility, as endometriosis or low ovarian reserve. Of them all, 137 women returned to use their oocytes.

Among several interesting findings we observed in this population, it is worth highlighting the age at vitrification and how it impacted on final outcomes. In our experience, most women are deciding for EFP at advanced age. Accordingly, 63% of them came to vitrify at ages between 37 and 40, additionally, a not inconsiderable 16.2% were aged ≥40 years old by the time of vitrification, while conversely, the vast minority were younger than 30 years of age [4]. As expectable, the age at vitrification had great impact on different outcomes related to the number of oocytes retrieved and the number of MII finally vitrified, oocytes' survival, pregnancy and live birth rates. Larger number of oocytes were either retrieved or vitrified in patients aged 35 years or younger when compared to patients older than 35 years. Furthermore, the lowest figures were observed in patients aged 40 years or older (5.1 (95% CI = 4.2–6.0) mean retrieved and 3.9 (95% CI = 2.6–5.0) mean MII vitrified).

As shown in Table 10.1 [4], survival was higher in the group of women aged ≤35 years (94.6% [95% CI = 91.9–97.3] vs. 82.4% [95% CI = 79.9–84.9]). The live birth rate per patient was statistically higher in younger patients when compared to the older ones (50% [95% CI = 32.7–67.3] vs. 22.9% [95% CI = 14.9–30.9]). Table 10.1-Panel II. shows the outcomes according to different subgroups of age showing the noticeable decrease in the live birth rate from the youngest category including women aged ≤29 years (100% [95% CI = 100–100]) to the oldest group of women aged 40–44 years (3.7% [95% CI = −3.4–10.8]).

The cumulative probability of having a child according to the number oocytes consumed by the statistical approach using Kaplan Meier was also assessed (Fig. 10.1) [4]. If women were 35 years or younger, we observed a huge difference in the cumulative live birth rate (CLBR) when using only five oocytes (15.4%) com-

Table 10.1 Clinical outcome according to age at vitrification

Age	N° patients	N° cycles	Survival rate	CPR/cycle	CPR/ET	OPR/cycle	OPR/ET	N° Live birth /patient
I. Survival and clinical outcome in patients aged ≤35 years and ≥36 years at vitrification								
≤35	32	41	257/272 (94.6)^{a}	24/41 (58.5)^{a}	24/39 (61.5)^{a}	21/41 (51.2)^{a}	21/39 (53.9)^{a}	16/32 (50)^{a}
≥36	105	150	750/910 (82.4)^{b}	47/150 (31.3)^{b}	47/118 (39.8)^{b}	27/150 (18.0)^{b}	27/118 (22.9)^{b}	24/105 (22.9)^{b}
Total	137	191	1007/1182 (85.2)	71/191 (37.1)	71/157 (45.2)	48/191 (25.1)	48/157 (30.5)	40/137 (29.2)
II. Survival and clinical outcome according to different groups of age at vitrification								
≤29	6	9	59/62 (94.5)^{a}	6/9 (66.6)^{a}	6/9 (66.6)^{a}	6/9 (66.6)^{a}	6/9 (66.6)^{a}	6/6 (100)^{a}
30–34	20	23	155/161 (96.1)^{a}	14/23 (60.9)^{a}	14/21 (66.7)^{a}	13/23 (56.5)^{a}	13/21 (61.9)^{a}	9/20 (45)^{b}
35–39	84	127	601/734 (81.8)^{b}	48/127 (37.8)^{b}	48/112 (42.9)^{b}	27/127 (21.3)^{b}	27 /112 (24.1)^{b}	24/84 (28.5)^{b}
≥40	27	32	192/225 (85.3)^{b}	3/32 (9.8)^{c}	3/15 (20)^{c}	2/32 (6.3)^{c}	2/15 (13.3)^{b}	1 (3.7)^{c}
Total	137	191	1007/1182 (85.2)	71/191 (37.1)	71/157 (45.2)	48/191 (25.1)	48/157 (30.5)	40/137 (29.2)

CPR clinical pregnancy rate, *OPR* ongoing pregnancy rate, *ET* embryo transfer

Different superscripts in the same column indicate statistical differences ($P < 0.05$). Includes embryo cryo-transfers. Cobo et al. Fertil Steril 105 [3]: 755–764 e758 [4]

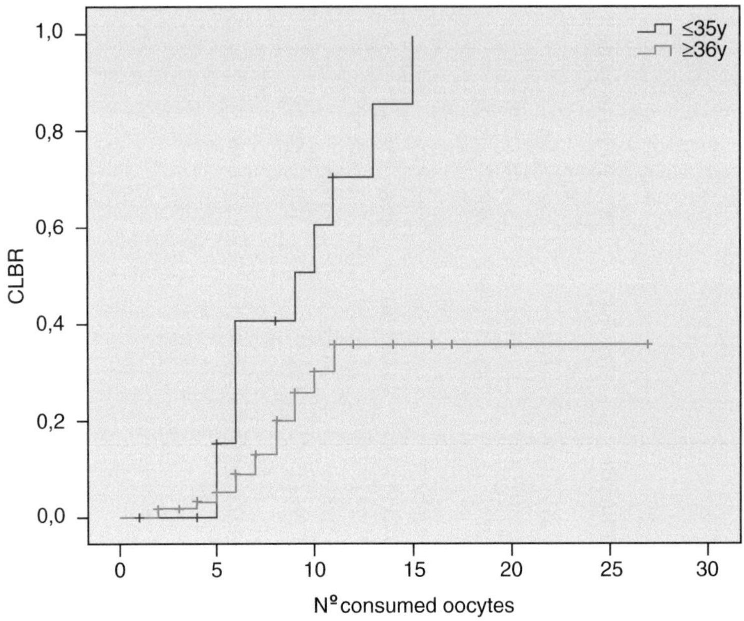

≤35 years old	
N° oocytes	**CLBR (IC95%)**
5	15,4 (-4.2-35.0)
8	40.8 (13.2-68.4)
9	50,6 (31.6-79.6)
10	60,5 (34.5-89.5)
15	85,2 (60.5-100)

≥36 years old	
N° oocytes	**CLBR (95% CI)**
5	5,1 (-0.6-10.7)
8	19,9 (8.7-31.1)
9	25.8 (12.7-38.9)
10	29,7 (15.2-34.2)
11	35,6 (18.4-52.8)

Fig. 10.1 CLBR according to age (≤35 and ≥36y) and number of oocytes consumed. Cobo et al. Fertil Steril 105 [3]: 755–764 e758 [4]

pared to employing eight (40.8%) which means an 8.4% increase in CLBR per additional oocyte. On the other hand, if they were 36 years or older using the same number of oocytes the increase in CLBR was considerably milder (from 5.1% CLBR using 5 oocytes to 19.9% when 8 oocytes were consumed, meaning an increase in CLBR of 4.9%). Moreover, the success rate achieved in the younger group (≤35 years) was twice the achieved in the older group of women aged ≥36 years (60.5% vs. 29.7% respectively) when 10 oocytes were used. With 15 oocytes the CLBR continue to increase in the ≤35 years group, whereas with the same number of oocytes the plateau was already reached in the group of women aged ≥36 years, meaning that at this point the success is independent from the number of oocytes used up. In light of this, we suggest that at least 8–10MII should be vitrified

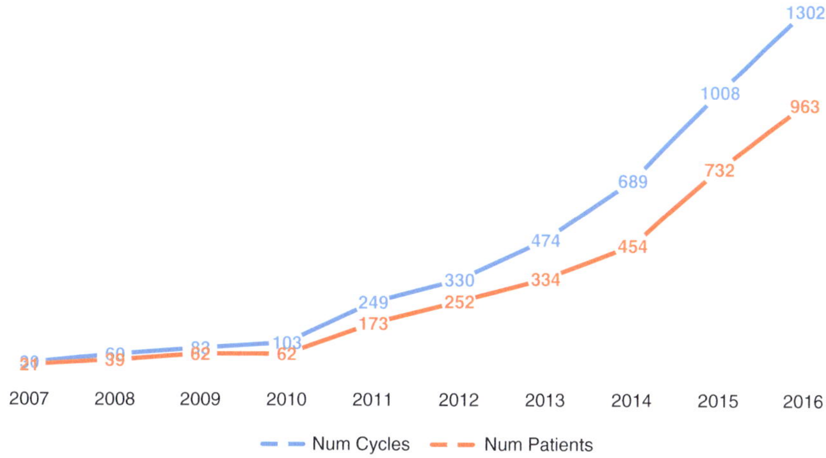

Fig. 10.2 Trends of the utilization of oocytes vitrification as a strategy for elective fertility preservation during the past 9 years. Number of patients and vitrification cycles are shown

to obtain a reasonable success rate. In women older than 36 years, numbers should be individualized along with the possibility of offering PGS.

All these findings have helped to consolidate the approach of oocytes vitrification in cases of elective fertility preservation, fact that has contributed to the increase in the number of women deciding for this strategy as a way to alleviate the pressure posed by their every particular circumstance. In accordance, the most recent analysis of our data on fertility preservation of for social reasons during the 9 years of this practice in our setting shows clear increasing trends in the application of oocytes vitrification for EFP (Fig. 10.2). A total of 3092 patients have conducted 4328 (1.4 ± 1.1) vitrification cycles for EFP from September 2007 to December 2016. Most of them had high educational level (74.8%), while the majority were heterosexual single women (77.9%). The remaining women were heterosexual married women (21.6%) and only 0.5% were homosexual.

Mean patients' age at vitrification was 37.2 ± 3.9 years old. As shown in Fig. 10.3, the great majority (73.6%) decided for oocytes vitrification between 35 and 40 years old, which is the age at which most women consult for AR treatments, due to the well-known age-related fertility decline. As shown in Fig. 10.4, among the 353 patients who have returned to use their oocytes nearly 80% vitrified at ages between 35 and 41 years. Additionally, shorter storage time was observed for patients older than 36 years old when compared to those aged 35 or lower (1.7 ± 0.6 vs. 2.9 ± 1.4 years of storage respectively). The debate is then served, since as we demonstrated earlier (Table 10.1) the efficiency in terms of live birth rate per patient is much lower in patients older than 36 years old and worsens dramatically at 40s [4]. In light of these findings, patients should be counsel to decide earlier for oocytes vitrification. However, another debate related to cost-effectiveness becomes relevant, being that recent data shows that egg banking for fertility preservation is more cost-effective in women under the age of 38 years [5, 6].

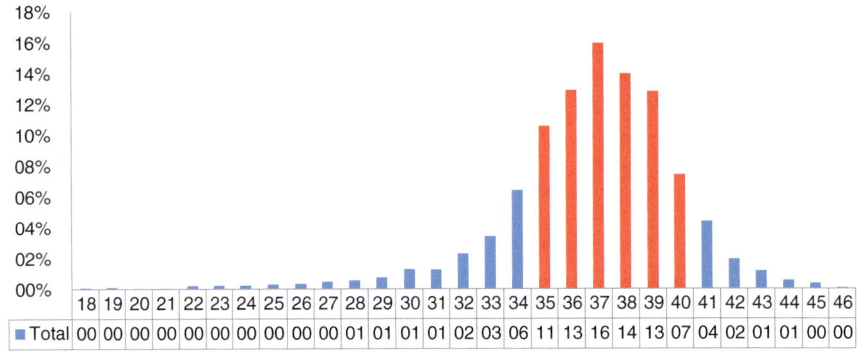

Fig. 10.3 Distribution of patients age at vitrification

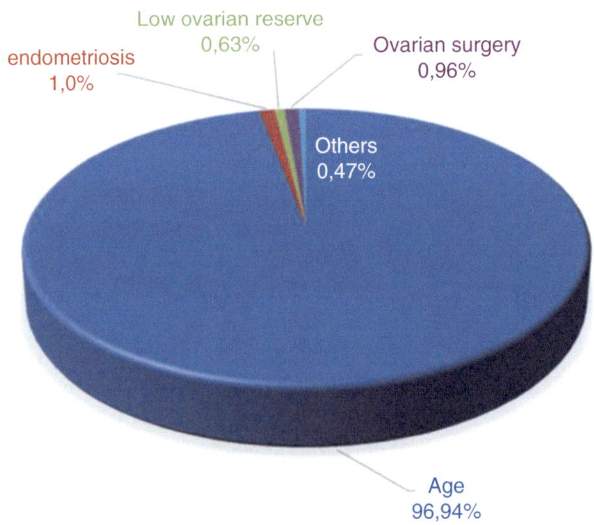

Fig. 10.4 Distribution of women who had returned to use their oocytes in the 9 years of EFP in our centers (2007–2016)

Although the two arguments are valid, we think that it is absolutely necessary to adequately inform the patients both the very young women, and enlightening them that the probability of using their cryo-stored eggs in the upcoming years is reduced, due to, in the future; their chance of natural conception could remain high. On the other hand, older women, who are more likely to use their cryo-savings, should be accurately informed about their reduced reproductive chances. Anyway, as we have demonstrated, a child can be achieved when oocytes were vitrified over 40s, making very difficult to set upper limits for applying the strategy.

Table 10.2 Clinical outcome after 9 years of applying elective fertility preservation (2007–2016)

Elective fertility preservation		
		IC95%
Patients returning	353	
Warming Cycles	373 (1.1 ± 0.05)	1.09–1.2
Mean warmed oocytes/patient	3245 (9.2 ± 4.8)	9.1–9.3
Survival rate	2641 (81.4)	81.1–82.7
Number of transfers	252 (71.4)	65.8–76.9
Mean embryos Transferred	384 (1.03 ± 0.8)	0.9–1.1
IR	36.7	31.4–43.4
CPR/transfer	116 (46.4)	40.3–52.6
OPR/transfer	85 (34.1)	28.3–40.0
N° Live Birth	63	
Cryotransfers of surplus embryos		
N° patients	81	
N° warming cycles	110 (1.4 ± 0.1)	1.3–1.4
N°ET	143 (1.8 ± 0.5)	1.7–1.9
N°Cryo transfers	106	
IR	35.7	27.9–43.6
CPR/transfer	49 (46.2)	36.7–55.7
OPR/transfer	32 (30.2)	21.5–38.9
N° Live Birth	21	
Total Live birth	84	
C Live birth rate/patient	23.8	19.4–28.2

Figure 10.4, shows the distribution of 3092 women who conducted EFP in our units during the period of 2007–2016. Table 10.2 shows a summary of clinical outcomes achieved when the 353 women returned to attempt pregnancy with their vitrified oocytes. A total of 3245 oocytes were warmed up (mean = 9.2 ± 4.8; 95% CI = 9.1–9.3). The overall survival rate was 81.4% (N = 2641 oocytes; 95% CI = 81.1–82.7). A number of 384 (mean per patient = 1.03 ± 0.8 95% CI = 0.9–1.1) embryos were transferred in 252 embryo transfers (mean per patient = 71.4; 95% CI = 65.8–76.9). Implantation rate was 36.7% (95% CI = 31.4–43.4) and clinical and ongoing pregnancy rates were 46.4% (95% CI = 40.3–52.6) and 34.1% (95% CI = 28.3–40.0) respectively. Sixty-three healthy babies were born.

A number of 81 patients who had surplus embryos for additional cryotransfers performed 110 embryo- warming cycles (mean/patient = 1.4 ± 0.1). A mean of 1.8 ± 0.5 embryos were transferred in 106 cryo-transfers (mean/patient = 1.3 ± 2.5) achieving 35.7% implantation rate. Cumulative Clinical and ongoing pregnancy rates considering fresh and all cryo-transfers were (53.6% and 40.8% respectively). Twenty-one babies were born from these cryo-transfers. The cumulative livebirth rate per patient was 23.8% (95% CI = 19.4–28.2), being higher in younger women (51.3% when patients vitrified at 35 years or earlier vs. 16.2% when they were older than 35 years at vitrification).

In conclusion, the efficiency of oocytes vitrification for save guarding fertility is currently a consolidated option that can be offered to women seeking an option to achieve motherhood in the future. However, we think it is mandatory to explain to women who seek EFP that oocyte cryo-storage is no insurance policy to secure future motherhood, but a means to increase the chances of having a biological child, and that these chances depend on age and on the number of oocytes stored. It is imperative that women are informed about the drop in the probability of success over the age of 35 years. The number of vitrified oocytes should be adjusted according to the patient's age in order to increase the probability of having a child, irrespectively of oocytes coming from one stimulation cycle or more. In cases of EFP, women should be encouraged to decide this option when younger than 35 years due to greater biological efficiency, although the strategy could be less cost-effective at younger ages.

Key Points

1. The clinical outcome with the use of vitrified oocytes is comparable to outcomes achieved with fresh oocytes
2. Currently, mostly women perform elective oocyte vitrification between the age of 35 and 40 years.
3. The efficiency in terms of live birth is much lower in patients performing oocyte vitrification after the age of 36 years and worsens dramatically after the age of 40.
4. Women who consider elective oocyte cryopreservation should be encouraged to do so before the age of 35, although this could be less cost-effective.
5. It remains important to counsel women that elective oocyte cryopreservation can increase future reproductive chances but cannot guarantee reproductive success.

References

1. Cobo A, Kuwayama M, Perez S, Ruiz A, Pellicer A, Remohi J. Comparison of concomitant outcome achieved with fresh and cryopreserved donor oocytes vitrified by the Cryotop method. Fertil Steril. 2008;89:1657–64.
2. Cobo A, Meseguer M, Remohi J, Pellicer A. Use of cryo-banked oocytes in an ovum donation programme: a prospective, randomized, controlled, clinical trial. Hum Reprod. 2010;25:2239–46.
3. Garcia-Velasco JA, Domingo J, Cobo A, Martinez M, Carmona L, Pellicer A. Five years' experience using oocyte vitrification to preserve fertility for medical and nonmedical indications. Fertil Steril. 2013;99:1994–9.
4. Cobo A, Garcia-Velasco JA, Coello A, Domingo J, Pellicer A, Remohi J. Oocyte vitrification as an efficient option for elective fertility preservation. Fertil Steril. 2016;105:755–64e8.
5. Mesen TB, Mersereau JE, Kane JB, Steiner AZ. Optimal timing for elective egg freezing. Fertil Steril. 2015;103:1551–6e1–4.
6. Waldby C. 'Banking time': egg freezing and the negotiation of future fertility. Cult Health Sex. 2015;17:470–82.

Chapter 11
Safety of Preventive Oocyte Cryopreservation

Shruti Parikh and Christophe Blockeel

Introduction

Developments in the discipline of reproductive medicine have been on a constant rise since its conception. Successful oocyte cryopreservation has been one such breakthrough, which has expanded the scope of treatment with assisted reproductive technology.

Initially, oocyte cryopreservation was restricted to use in cancer patients undergoing gonadotoxic treatment to conserve their fertility. However, over the recent years, oocyte freezing is also being popularly applied for non-medical indications wherein women are offered the chance to freeze their oocytes in anticipation of age related fertility decline for use at a later date; thus, extending the scope of IVF from a medical to social practice [1–3]. The use of ART procedures in normal healthy women has further emphasized the need for simpler and more patient friendly stimulation protocols.

Ovarian Stimulation

Ovarian stimulation protocols aim to achieve multi-follicular growth without causing a premature rise in LH. Exogenous gonadotropins administered during folliculogenesis maintain the FSH levels above the threshold, prolonging the duration that

S. Parikh
Shruti Nursing Home, Mumbai, India

C. Blockeel (✉)
Centre for Reproductive Medicine, Universitair Ziekenhuis Brussel, Vrije Universiteit Brussel, 101 Laarbeeklaan, Brussel 1090, Belgium
e-mail: Christophe.Blockeel@uzbrussel.be

© Springer International Publishing Switzerland 2018

D. Stoop (ed.), *Preventing Age Related Fertility Loss*,
DOI 10.1007/978-3-319-14857-1_11

the *FSH window* is open. This interferes with the natural process of dominant follicle selection and results in simultaneous growth of a cohort of follicles [4].

In the early twentieth century, factors with similar actions to anterior pituitary gonadotropins were discovered from urine of pregnant and postmenopausal women. By 1940, it was known that these factors were required for growth of follicles, but the use of these extracts was limited due to the development of severe antibody reactions [5]. In 1947, human menopausal gonadotropin (hMG) was created by using extraction methods to reduce the content of protein impurities. Despite this, the pharmacologically active content was only <5% having equal FSH: LH bioactivity [4]. With further purification, the LH component kept reducing and hCG was added to the preparation to restore the lost LH bioactivity. Thus highly purified hMG (HP-hMG) contains more hCG compared to uhMG; reduced protein impurities make HP-hMG safe for subcutaneous administration as well [6]. The advent of monoclonal antibodies reactive to FSH, allowed for the recovery of only FSH component with negligible LH activity and lesser protein impurities (uFSH) along with its highly purified version HP-uFSH [7].

The ever growing demand for gonadotropins was fulfilled with their in *vitro* production using recombinant DNA technology in mammalian cell culture systems (recFSH, recLH, rechCG) [8]. These recombinant products have added benefits of improved purity due to which they can be administered by protein weight (filled by Mass) rather than bioactivity, increasing the batch-to-batch consistency of the gonadotropin injections [8, 9].

Dosage of gonadotropins (hMG and rec FSH being most frequently used) are individualized but usually commenced in a dose range between 150 and 300 IU. There is not much evidence regarding the benefit of dosage adjustment mid-cycle [10]. A meta-analysis in 2008 has shown better pregnancy and live birth rates in a GnRH agonist setting for hMG versus rec FSH [11]; no difference in outcome was demonstrated in the GnRH antagonist protocol [12, 13]. The largest meta-analysis to date (2010) comparing stimulation with hMG versus rec FSH in fresh cycles have shown that even though rec FSH is associated with retrieval of larger number of oocytes with significantly lower dosage of gonadotropins consumed, there is no significant difference in the baseline adjusted pregnancy rates [14]. The Cochrane database (2011) showed similar efficacy with respect to the two gonadotropins in both the GnRH analogue protocols [14, 15].

The most recent gonadotropin developed is long acting FSH (Corifollitropin alpha) generated using site directed mutagenesis and gene transfer techniques to attach the carboxy terminal peptide (CTP) of β hCG subunit to the β chain of recombinant FSH molecule [16]. It has a similar action to rec FSH interacting with the FSH receptor and is devoid of LH activity. The CTP component containing 4 O-linked oligosaccharides gives it a prolonged half-life compared to rec FSH [17]. Thus a single bolus could induce and sustain the growth of multiple follicles similar to 150 IU of recFSH given daily for 7 days making it suitable for IVF cycles. Due to its pharmacokinetic profile, the use of corifollitropin alpha can eliminate the need for daily subcutaneous injections simplifying the stimulation process and reducing patient discomfort [18, 19]. Multiple dose finding studies comparing the efficacy of a single bolus of corifollitropin alpha versus daily rec FSH have proved corifollitropin alpha to be equally effective with respect to the number of oocytes collected and ongoing pregnancy rates [18–22]. Higher incidence of OHSS was found emphasizing caution in high responders and women with polycystic ovaries [19].

GnRH Analogues

The supra-physiological rise in the level of serum estradiol associated with multi-follicular development may cause a premature surge in LH and thus trigger premature luteinisation in the mature follicles or atresia in the immature ones resulting in cycle cancellation [23–25]. The use of GnRH analogues in stimulation protocols to prevent pituitary LH surge have significantly benefited IVF outcomes [4].

GnRH agonists were originally developed with the goal of treating anovulation; however, this soon changed to pituitary desensitization with the understanding of their mechanism of action. They bind to the GnRH receptors at the level of the pituitary causing an initial flare-up in gonadotropin levels followed by a decrease in the gonadal function. Prolonged occupation of the receptors causes desensitization due to their clustering and internalization resulting in pituitary quiescence (7–14 days) [26]. Their use was associated with significant reduction in the cycle cancellation rate occurring due to premature LH surge as well as better scheduling of oocyte retrievals [27]. GnRH agonists have been used for over 30 years in IVF with many studies comparing the various protocols for their administration.

The long protocol, which is the most commonly used GnRH agonist protocol, achieves pituitary quiescence before the start of stimulation. Agonists are administered from the luteal phase of the previous cycle and stimulation is commenced only after complete pituitary down regulation is achieved. Due to their initial flare up effect it takes about 2 weeks for complete pituitary block, which causes significantly prolonged stimulation cycles [28]. There are reports of severe hypo-estrogenic state due to prolonged down-regulation in some women associated with symptoms of hot flushes, sweating, weight gain, mood changes, etc. Also commencing treatment in the luteal phase poses a risk of inadvertent stimulation during pregnancy and is also associated with the chance of ovarian cyst formation, both of which can be reduced by pretreatment with oral contraceptive (OC) pills [29, 30].

In the short GnRH agonist protocol, GnRH agonists are started a day prior to stimulation. The initial flare thus coincides with the rise in FSH, theoretically benefitting multi-follicular growth. Follicular maturation is usually achieved by the 12th day of the cycle which is adequate for pituitary desensitization, thus premature LH surge is prevented [31].

A meta-analysis comparing the short and long GnRH agonist protocols shows a clear benefit in terms of oocyte retrieval and pregnancy rate with use of the long protocol, however, the long protocol is associated with significantly higher consumption of gonadotropins [32]. The long luteal (mid luteal) GnRH agonist administration is associated with the best oocyte retrieval rate compared with early/late luteal or follicular start of the agonist [33, 34]. Optimal scheduling of oocyte retrieval is a possible advantage with the long agonist protocol, as exogenous stimulation can be delayed after pituitary quiescence without an impact on IVF outcome [35, 36].

Though introduced a while ago, GnRH antagonists have only recently been accepted for use in IVF cycles. Their limited popularity arose due to an initial Cochrane analysis, which showed lower chances of clinical pregnancy with antagonist as compared to agonist use [37]. However, there was no difference in the live birth rate, but this was not studied.

Unlike the agonist, the antagonists have a straightforward mechanism of action; they competitively bind with the GnRH receptor causing an instantaneous fall in pituitary production of gonadotropins. This mechanism allows for their administration only when LH surge is expected (cycle day 5—day 7 onwards) eliminating the need for their prolonged administration prior to stimulation [38]. Their rapid action drastically reduces the duration of ovarian stimulation and total gonadotropin consumption. Lack of initial stimulatory effect eliminates the risk of cyst formation with the use of the GnRH antagonist. Also, unlike the GnRH agonist there are no acute periods of hypo-estrogenaemia with the use of GnRH antagonist thus symptoms like hot flushes, mood swings etc. are not associated with their use [39].

GnRH antagonist action is dose dependent, mediated on balance between endogenous GnRH and the administered GnRH antagonist; thus much higher doses of antagonist compared to GnRH agonist are required to block endogenous LH [40]. Fixed day 6 administration of GnRH antagonist appears to be superior to the flexible protocol (administration when follicle > 14 mm size), however due to small risk of LH escape before start of the GnRH antagonist, clinicians are now favouring earlier day 5 start versus day 6 [37, 41]. The daily dose administration (0.25 mg of Ganirelix/Cetrorelix) is preferred to the fixed single dose (3 mg of Cetrorelix), though studies have shown no difference between the two with respect to clinical pregnancy rate [42, 43].

Several studies comparing the long GnRH agonist and the GnRH antagonist cycles are now published. The meta-analysis and systemic review by Kolibianakis et al. (2006) shows no difference in live birth rate with regard to the GnRH analogue used to suppress the LH surge [41]. Recent Cochrane meta-analyses (2011–2016) have also shown similar efficacy in both groups [44, 45]. Also no difference has been demonstrated in terms of embryo or endometrium quality between the two analogues [46–49]. Antagonist cycles are associated with slightly higher chances of premature LH surge, however in all the cases the surge occurred before the start of the GnRH antagonist indicating the need for earlier start of the antagonist (day 5 start instead of day 6) [50].

Non-significant higher live birth rate and higher oocyte yield exists with GnRH agonist however such differences are negligible especially due to the non-outcome benefits of the GnRH antagonists which have made IVF stimulation cycles simpler and more patient friendly [51].

Ovulation Trigger

Due to the unpredictability of LH rise during stimulation, hCG has been uniformly used as a final oocyte maturation trigger in IVF cycles. hCG binds to the LH/hCG receptor and in the presence of pre-ovulatory follicles causes granulosa cell luteinisation with subsequent progesterone production, resumption of meiosis, oocyte maturation followed by follicle rupture 36–40 h later [52, 53].

However, hCG differs from the physiological surge as it does not induce FSH rise; also, it has a longer serum half-life compared to LH. Hence, its administration is associated with a sustained luteotropic effect with multiple corpora lutea development and supraphysiological steroid levels [54], increasing the risk of developing ovarian hyperstimulation [55].

In order to minimize the patient's burden and risk of complications, recent studies are focusing on the use of GnRH agonist to induce final oocyte maturation. When used in a GnRH antagonist setting, the GnRH agonist displaces the antagonist from its pituitary receptor, which causes a surge in LH and FSH levels (flare effect); followed by down regulation of the receptor [56]. Like the physiological mid-cycle surge, GnRH agonist trigger induces FSH rise as well, which is proposed to have a role in completion of oocyte meiosis, cumulus expansion and induction of LH receptors on the granulosa cells [57–61]. However, the LH surge following agonist trigger has only 2 phases (~24–36 h) and is of a much shorter duration resulting in deficient luteal gonadotropin levels [54, 62]. The early corpus luteum demise results in reduced secretion of vasoactive peptides and is thus associated with reduced risk of OHSS. Studies have shown that GnRH agonist trigger is associated with better patient comfort with lesser abdominal bloating due to reduced ovarian volumes, reduced fluid in cul de sac and earlier onset of menses [63–65].

GnRH agonist trigger used in fresh cycles has shown to have an impact on pregnancy outcome due to early luteolysis. However, this deficient luteal phase affects only the endometrium without any effect on the oocyte maturation and/or embryo quality, as seen in oocyte donation cycles [66–69], implying that GnRH agonist trigger can safely be used in segmented IVF cycles (cryopreservation of oocytes) [70].

The differences between hCG and GnRH agonist as a trigger are shown in Fig. 11.1.

However, an important question still remains- "Is the GnRH agonist trigger really the Holy Grail?"

	hCG	GnRH agonist
Mechanism	Biologic similarity to LH	GnRH antagonist displacement[53,60]
FSH surge	No	Yes (flare-up)[53,60]
Luteotropic effect	Sustained (present up to 6 days after 500IU)	Shorter70[70,71,72]
Luteal phase steroids	High	Closer to physiologic ranges[70,71,72]

Fig. 11.1 Differences between hCG and GnRH agonist trigger

OHSS

The ovarian hyperstimulation syndrome is a serious, potentially lethal complication of IVF, with an incidence ranging from 0.1 to 2% for severe cases to as high as 22% for mild ones [74]. It is characterized by bilateral enlargement of ovaries with an extravascular fluid shift secondary to increased vascular permeability. hCG is known to play a central role in its development and thus recent trends in ART practice are shifting towards use of GnRH agonist for final maturation trigger.

The risk of OHSS is not completely eliminated with the use of the GnRH agonist trigger. Some cases of early onset OHSS have been reported despite the use of GnRH agonist for oocyte final maturation (without any luteal phase medication) [65, 75–77] Case reports have pointed to a high AMH in their patients, which could be a red flag for differentiating women who may develop OHSS despite GnRH agonist trigger. However, larger studies are required to prove the association of high AMH with this risk.

Genetic predisposition for development of OHSS exists like alleles of FSH receptor, estrogen receptors, aromatase genes, vascular endothelial growth factor gene variation and LH–chorionic gonadotropin genetic variation. However, these are far from complete as a case report by Santos-Ribeiro et al. has shown development of OHSS in a patient with no definitive genetic predisposition analysed by whole exome sequencing [65]. Thus, detailed genetic analysis is required in extreme severe OHSS cases to better understand the pathophysiology of OHSS and genetic predisposition in women who develop this following GnRH agonist trigger.

Adnexal Torsion

Adnexal torsion is a well recognised emergency of the hyper-stimulated ovary more common in first and second trimesters of pregnancy, with a lower incidence of around 0.2% in oocyte donors [78] Prompt diagnosis is the key to ovarian salvage; may be more than often delayed due to similarity of symptoms with ovarian hyper-stimulation like abdominal distension and abdominal tenderness. Simple untwisting (detorsion) of the adnexa to restore blood supply is associated with good prognosis if the accident is picked up early. Colour doppler can help in early diagnosis with finding of decreased diastolic blood flow [79]. Reducing OHSS and high degree of suspicion in women who develop ovarian hyper-response are required to reduce the incidence of adnexal accidents and for the conservative management of torsion.

Suboptimal Response

A concern arising with the use of GnRH agonist as ovulation trigger is the suboptimal response observed in a subset of patients who do not respond with an adequate endogenous LH surge. This can be expected from women with hypothalamic-hypogonadic amenorrhoea. However, women with regular menses but having a down-regulated hypothalamic-pituitary axis have shown to be at a greater risk of a suboptimal response [80]. These patients characteristically have very low LH and FSH at the start of the cycle, requiring more exogenous gonadotropins and having longer duration of stimulation. A suboptimal responder phenotype has been identified—younger, low BMI, more common in oocyte donors, long term OC pill users [80]. Screening patients with pre-trigger LH values <0.5 IU/L may help identify women likely to elicit a suboptimal response to GnRH agonist trigger [80]. Also, monitoring of post trigger (12 h)serum LH levels could serve as an indicator of suboptimal response following GnRH agonist trigger and appropriate action could be taken (re-trigger with hCG) to avoid retrieval of immature oocytes. Although no fixed value of LH or progesterone is defined for inadequate response, studies have shown that patients with failed maturation had a post trigger LH <15 IU/L [56].

Ideal Timing of Triggering Final Oocyte Maturation

In regular IVF patients, the timing of trigger is crucial in a GnRH antagonist protocol cycle as studies have shown that delay in the trigger after 3 follicles of >17 mm diameter is associated with decline in pregnancy rates. This is probably due to rise in the progesterone level, which affects the endometrium causing premature decidualization thus, lowering the implantation rates [81]. Prolongation of the follicular phase however does not seem to have any adverse effect on the oocyte quality nor cleavage rate in the embryo as reported in a study on oocyte donation cycles [82]. Thus, delay in trigger during segmentation IVF cycles may be beneficial by improving the number of mature oocytes retrieved [82]. However, delaying the final maturation trigger (till 3 follicles > 20/22 mm) without any adverse outcomes in segmented IVF cycles, still needs to be established by further studies.

Complications Related to the Oocyte Retrieval Procedure

Minor complications like vaginal bleeding are reported in 8.6% of oocyte donors undergoing oocyte pick-up procedure and can be managed conservatively with vaginal tamponade and rarely sutures [83, 84].

Intra-abdominal bleeding secondary to bleeding from ruptured follicle or injury to surrounding blood vessels and ovarian capsular bleeding is potentially more dangerous but not so common with an incidence of around 0.02–0.3% [83, 85–87].

Pelvic infections in patients undergoing IVF cycles was reported at 0.01–0.6% and is expected to be lower in oocyte donors due to lower incidence of pelvic inflammatory disease, hydrosalpinges and endometriomas in these women. Empirical use of antibiotics is not recommended; their use can be restricted to women with the above mentioned risk factors of infection [83–86, 88, 89].

Oncological Risks

Female cancers like breast cancer, uterine cancer or ovarian cancer have a known multifactorial etiology with hormonal factors playing an important role in development of most of these cancers [90]. Thus the safety of short duration of supraphysiological hormone levels during IVF with regard to the potential oncological risks needs to be addressed.

A meta-analysis in 2013 including a total of 746,455 patients has shown an increased risk of ovarian cancer development in patients undergoing IVF treatment (RR-1.59) [91]. Similar findings were published in another meta-analysis done in the same year [92]. However, the increased risk in these patients existed only when comparing with the general population. The risks was not present when comparing patients undergoing IVF with other sub-fertile women. These findings were also reported in a recent analysis in 2015, showing an association between IVF treatment and risk of developing ovarian cancer even after cofounding factors like maternal age and obesity were controlled [93].

Unopposed estradiol exposure is a known risk factor for the development of endometrial cancer and thus as one would expect an increased risk of uterine cancer with the use of gonadotropins and more than 6 cycles of fertility treatment have been reported by a Danish study in 2009 [94]. Similar association between uterine cancer and IVF treatment have been reported in a study by Lerner Geva et al. (with a 30 year follow-up period) and another meta-analysis done in 2015 [93, 95]. However no association was found between risk of developing uterine cancer and ovulation induction [95].

Multiple meta-analyses have evaluated the risk of breast cancer subsequent to IVF treatment and they did not reveal any association between the use of fertility drugs for IVF and future risk of breast cancer [93, 96]. However, higher absolute dense volumes on mammogram were reported in women treated with controlled ovarian stimulation suggesting need for continued monitoring of cancer risk in women undergoing ovarian stimulation [97].

However, most studies to date evaluate the oncological risks among infertile women undergoing IVF stimulation. Multiple factors causing infertility in women themselves independently affect the risks of female oncological cancers. Thus further studies in healthy women undergoing stimulation for oocyte freezing or oocyte donation are required.

Effects on Ovarian Reserve and Future Fertility

Studies with oocyte donors have reported 5–9.6% incidence of fertility issues in donor patients requiring further treatment [98, 99]. Both studies evaluated the short term effects on fertility. Further trials studying the potential long term fertility effects of IVF stimulation and oocyte puncture need to be evaluated. Another trial comparing serum AMH levels in oocyte donor patients has shown no significant drop in the serum AMH levels after repetitive oocyte punctures for oocyte donation, again emphasising the potential lack of any immediate effects on fertility [100].

To conclude, ART stimulation is an elective procedure on apparently healthy women and thus it is of vital importance that the stimulation is simplified with the exclusion of the risks as much as possible. Despite the advances in IVF practices, OHSS still remains the most lethal iatrogenic complication following stimulation and thus is a cause of anxiety for most of the clinicians [101]. Efforts to improve outcomes and reduce the risks are being made and one such modification was the introduction of the GnRH antagonist protocol during the stimulation cycle. Their use is associated with simpler stimulation cycles and reduced side effects with a similar outcome in terms of live birth rates as compared to GnRH agonists. They also allow for the use of GnRH agonist to trigger the final oocyte maturation, which has significantly dropped the risks of developing OHSS. However, as mentioned previously, OHSS is not completely eliminated with their use. Also there is a small subset of patients who develop an inadequate response to the GnRH agonist trigger. Thus, maturation trigger with GnRH agonist still deserves further scrutiny with well-designed randomised controlled trials.

Key Message

1. The GnRH antagonist protocol is the first treatment of choice for oocyte cryopreservation
2. The use of GnRH agonist for trigger in a GnRH antagonist cycle dramatically reduces the risks of OHSS development; however the risk is not completely eliminated.
3. Caution is needed with regard to the suboptimal response after the GnRH agonist trigger.
4. Further studies concerning oncological risks of ovarian stimulation are urgently needed.

References

1. Sanchez-Serrano M, Crespo J, Mirabet V, Cobo AC, Escriba MJ, Simon C, Pellicer A. Twins born after transplantation of ovarian cortical tissue and oocyte vitrification. Fertil Steril. 2010;93(1):268.e11–3.
2. Cobo A, Domingo J, Perez S, Crespo J, Remohi J, Pellicer A. Vitrification, an effective new approach to oocyte banking in healthy women, could be applied in cancer patients to preserve their fertility. Clin Transl Oncol. 2008;10:268–73.
3. Homburg R, Van der Veen F, Silber SJ. Oocyte vitrification-women's emancipation set in stone. Fertil Steril. 2009;91(Suppl 4):1319–20.
4. Macklon NS, Stouffer RL, Giudice LC, Fauser BCJM. The science behind 24 years of ovarian stimulation for in vitro fertilization. Endocr Rev. 2010;27(2):170–207.
5. Lunenfeld B. Historical perspectives in gonadotropin therapy. Hum Reprod Update. 2004;10:453–67.
6. Al-Inany HG, bou-Setta AM, Aboulghar MA, et al. Highly purified hMG achieves better pregnancy rates in IVF cycles but not ICSI cycles compared with rec FSH: a meta-analysis. Gynecol Endocrinol. 2009;25:372–8.
7. Le Cotonnec JY, Porchet HC, Beltrami V, Howles C. Comparative pharmacokinetics of two urinary human follicle stimulating hormone preparations in healthy female and male volunteers. Hum Reprod. 1993;8(10):1604–11.
8. Fauser BC. Developments in human recombinant follicle stimulating hormone technology: are we going in the right direction? Hum Reprod. 1998;13(Suppl 3):36–46.
9. Keene JL, Matzuk MM, Otani T, Fauser BC, Galway AB, Hsueh AJ, Boime I. Expression of biologically active human follitropin in Chinese hamster ovary cells. J Biol Chem. 1989;264:4769–75.
10. Van Hooff MH, Alberda AT, Huisman GJ, Zeilmaker GH, Leerentveld RA. Doubling the human menopausal gonadotrophin dose in the course of an in-vitro fertilization treatment cycle in low responders: a randomized study. Hum Reprod. 1993;8:369–73.
11. Al-Inany H, Abou-Setta A, Aboulghar M, Mansour R, Serour G. Efficacy and safety of human menopausal gonadotropins versus recombinant FSH: a meta-analysis. Reprod Biomed Online. 2008;16(1):81–8.
12. Coomarasamy A, Afnan M, Cheema D, Van der Veen F, Bossuyt P, Van Wely M. Urinary hMG versus recombinant FSH for controlled ovarian hyper stimulation following an agonist long down-regulation protocol in IVF or ICSI treatment: a systematic review and meta-analysis. Hum Reprod. 2008;23(2):310–5.
13. Bosch E, Vidal C, Labarta E, Simon C, Remohi J, Pellicer A. Highly purified hMG versus recombinant FSH in ovarian hyper stimulation with GnRH antagonists-a randomized study. Hum Reprod. 2008;23(10):2346–51.

14. Lehert P, Schertz JC, Ezcurra D. Recombinant human follicle-stimulating hormone produces more oocytes with a lower total dose per cycle in assisted reproductive technologies compared with highly purified human menopausal gonadotrophin: a meta-analysis. Reprod Biol Endocrinol. 2010;8:112.
15. Westergaard LW, Bossuyt PM, Van der Veen F, van Wely M. Human menopausal gonadotropin versus recombinant follicle stimulation hormone for ovarian stimulation in assisted reproductive cycles. Cochrane Database Syst Rev. 2011;(2):CD003973.
16. Fares FA, Suganuma N, Nishimori K, LaPolt PS, Hsueh AJ, Boime I. Design of a long acting follitropin agonist by fusing the C-terminal sequence of the chorionic gonadotropin beta subunit to the follitropin beta subunit. Proc Natl Acad Sci U S A. 1992;89:4304–8.
17. Boime I, Ben-Menahem D. Glycoprotein hormone structure-function and analog design. Recent Prog Horm Res. 1999;54:271–88.
18. Fauser BC, Mannaerts BM, Devroey P, Leader A, Boime I, Baird DT. Advances in recombinant DNA technology: corifollitropin alfa, a hybrid molecule with sustained follicle-stimulating activity and reduced injection frequency. Hum Reprod Update. 2009;15:309–21.
19. Devroey P, Boostanfar R, Koper NP, Mannaerts BM, Ijzerman-Boon PC, Fauser BC, ENGAGE Investigators. A double-blind, non-inferiority RCT comparing corifollitropin alfa and recombinant FSH during the first seven days of ovarian stimulation using a GnRH antagonist protocol. Hum Reprod. 2009;24(12):3063–72.
20. Corifollitropin alfa Ensure Study Group. Corifollitropin alfa for ovarian stimulation in IVF: a randomized trial in lower-body-weight women. Reprod Biomed Online. 2010;21(1):66–76.
21. Mahmoud Youssef MA, Van WM, Aboulfoutouh I, El-Khyat W, van der Veen F, Al-Inany H. Is there a place for corifollitropin alfa in IVF/ICSI cycles? A systematic review and meta-analysis. Fertil Steril. 2012;97(4):876–85.
22. Fatemi HM, Blockeel C, Devroey P. Ovarian stimulation: today and tomorrow. Curr Pharm Biotechnol. 2012;13(3):392–7.
23. Fatemi H, Oberye J, Popovic-Todorovic B, Witjes H, Manaerts B, Devroey P. Corifollitropin alfa in a long GnRH agonist protocol: proof of concept trial. Fertil Steril. 2010;94(5):1992–24.
24. Hillier SG. Current concepts of the roles of follicle stimulating hormone and luteinizing hormone in folliculogenesis. Hum Reprod. 1994;9(2):188–91.
25. Chappel SC, Howles C. Reevaluation of the roles of luteinizing hormone and follicle-stimulating hormone in the ovulatory process. Hum Reprod. 1991;6(9):1206–12.
26. Conn PM, Crowley Jr WF. Gonadotropin-releasing hormone and its analogs. Annu Rev Med. 1994;45:391–405.
27. Smitz J, Devroey P, Camus M, Deschacht J, Khan I, Staessen C, Van Waesberghe L, Wisanto A, Van Steirteghem AC. The luteal phase and early pregnancy after combined GnRH-agonist/HMG treatment for superovulation in IVF or GIFT. Hum Reprod. 1988;3:585–90.
28. Barbieri RL, Hornstein MD. Assisted reproduction—in vitro fertilization success is improved by ovarian stimulation with exogenous gonadotropins and pituitary suppression with gonadotropin releasing hormone analogues. Endocr Rev. 1999;20:249–52.
29. Biljan MM, Mahutte NG, Dean N, Hemmings R, Bissonnette F, Tan SL. Pretreatment with an oral contraceptive is effective in reducing the incidence of functional ovarian cyst formation during pituitary suppression by gonadotropin-releasing hormone analogues. J Assist Reprod Genet. 1998;15(10):599–604.
30. Damario MA, Barmat L, Liu HC, Davis OK, Rosenwaks Z. Dual suppression with oral contraceptives and gonadotrophin releasing-hormone agonists improves in-vitro fertilization outcome in high responder patients. Hum Reprod. 1997;12(11):2359–65.
31. Smitz J, Devroey P, Van Steirteghem AC. Endocrinology in luteal phase and implantation. Br Med Bull. 1990;46:709–19.
32. Daya S. Gonadotropin releasing hormone agonist protocols for pituitary desensitization in in vitro fertilization and gamete intrafallopian transfer cycles. Cochrane Database Syst Rev. 2000;(2):CD001299.
33. Pellicer A, Simon C, Miro F, Castellvi RM, Ruiz A, Ruiz M, Perez M, Bonilla-Musoles F. Ovarian response and outcome of in-vitro fertilization in patients treated with gonadotro-

phin releasing hormone analogues in different phases of the menstrual cycle. Hum Reprod. 1989;4:285–9.

34. San Roman GA, Surrey ES, Judd HL, Kerin JF. A prospective randomized comparison of luteal phase versus concurrent follicular phase initiation of gonadotropin-releasing hormone agonist for in vitro fertilization. Fertil Steril. 1992;58:744–9.
35. Chang SY, Lee CL, Wang ML, Hu ML, Lai YM, Chang MY, Soong YK. No detrimental effects in delaying initiation of gonadotropin administration after pituitary desensitization with gonadotropin releasing hormone agonist. Fertil Steril. 1993;59:183–6.
36. Dimitry ES, Oskarsson T, Conaghan J, Margara R, Winston RM. Beneficial effects of a 24 h delay in human chorionic gonadotrophin administration during in-vitro fertilization treatment cycles. Hum Reprod. 1991;6:944–6.
37. Al-Inany HG, Abou-Setta AM, Aboulghar M. Gonadotrophin-releasing hormone antagonists for assisted conception. Cochrane Database Syst Rev. 2006;3:CD001750.
38. Klingmüller D, Schepke M, Enzweiler C, Bidlingmaier F. Hormonal responses to the new potent GnRH antagonist Cetrorelix. Acta Endocrinol. 1993;128(1):15–8.
39. Varney NR, Syrop C, Kubu CS, Struchen M, Hahn S, Franzen K. Neuropsychologic dysfunction in women following leuprolide acetate induction of hypoestrogenism. J Assist Reprod Genet. 1993;10(1):53–7.
40. Reissmann T, Felberbaum R, Diedrich K, Engel J, Comaru-Schally AM, Schally AV. Development and applications of luteinizing hormone-releasing hormone antagonists in the treatment of infertility: an overview. Hum Reprod. 1995;10(8):1974–81.
41. Kolibianakis EM, Collins J, Tarlatzis BC, Devroey P, Diedrich K, Griesinger G. Among patients treated for IVF with gonadotrophins and GnRH analogues, is the probability of live birth dependent on the type of analogue used? A systematic review and meta-analysis. Hum Reprod Update. 2006;12(6):651–71.
42. Diedrich K, Diedrich C, Santos E, Zoll C, al-Hasani S, Reissmann T, Krebs D, Klingmüller D. Suppression of the endogenous luteinizing hormone surge by the gonadotrophin-releasing hormone antagonist Cetrorelix during ovarian stimulation. Hum Reprod. 1994;9(5):788–91.
43. Lee TH, Wu MY, Chen HF, Chen MJ, Ho HN, Yang YS. Ovarian response and follicular development for single-dose and multiple-dose protocols for gonadotropin-releasing hormone antagonist administration. Fertil Steril. 2005;83(6):1700–7.
44. Al-Inany HG, Youssef MA, Aboulghar M, Broekmans F, Sterrenburg M, Smit J, Abou-Setta AM. GnRH antagonists are safer than agonists: an update of a Cochrane review. Hum Reprod Update. 2011;17(4):435.
45. Al-Inany HG, Youssef MA, Ayeleke RO, Brown J, Lam WS, Broekmans FJ. Gonadotrophin-releasing hormone antagonists for assisted reproductive technology. Cochrane Database Syst Rev. 2016;4:CD001750.
46. Kol S, Lightman A, Hillensjo T, Devroey P, Fauser B, Tarlatzis B, Mannaerts B, Itskovitz-Eldor J. High doses of gonadotrophin-releasing hormone antagonist in in-vitro fertilization cycles do not adversely affect the outcome of subsequent freeze-thaw cycles. Hum Reprod. 1999;14(9):2242–4.
47. Seelig AS, Al-Hasani S, Katalinic A, Schöpper B, Sturm R, Diedrich K, Ludwig M. Comparison of cryopreservation outcome with gonadotropin-releasing hormone agonists or antagonists in the collecting cycle. Fertil Steril. 2002;77(3):472–5.
48. Zikopoulos K, Kolibianakis EM, Camus M, Tournaye H, Van den Abbeel E, Joris H, Van Steirteghem A, Devroey P. Duration of gonadotropin-releasing hormone antagonist administration does not affect the outcome of subsequent frozen-thawed cycles. Fertil Steril. 2004;81(2):473–5.
49. Simon C, Oberyé J, Bellver J, Vidal C, Bosch E, Horcajadas JA, Murphy C, Adams S, Riesewijk A, Mannaerts B, Pellicer A. Similar endometrial development in oocyte donors treated with either high- or standard-dose GnRH antagonist compared to treatment with a GnRH agonist or in natural cycles. Hum Reprod. 2005;20(12):3318–27.
50. Kolibianakis EM, Albano C, Camus M, Tournaye H, Van Steirteghem AC, Devroey P. Initiation of gonadotropin-releasing hormone antagonist on day 1 as compared to day 6 of stimulation:

effect on hormonal levels and follicular development in in vitro fertilization cycles. J Clin Endocrinol Metab. 2003;88(12):5632–7.
51. Tarlatzis BC, Fauser BC, Kolibianakis EM, Diedrich K, Rombauts L, Devroey P. GnRH antagonists in ovarian stimulation for IVF. Hum Reprod Update. 2006;12(4):333–40.
52. Kessler M, Reddy M, Shah R, Bahl O. Structures of N- glycosidic carbohydrate units of human chorionic gonadotropin. J Biol Chem. 1979;254:7901–8.
53. Kyle CV, Griffin J, Jarrett A, Odell WD. Inability to demonstrate an ultrashort loop feedback mechanism for luteinizing hormone in humans. J Clin Endocrinol Metab. 1989;69(1):170–6.
54. Itskovitz J, Boldes R, Levron J, Erlik Y, Kahana L, Brandes J. Induction of preovulatory luteinizing hormone surge and prevention of ovarian hyperstimulation syndrome by gonadotropin releasing hormone agonist. Fertil Steril. 1991;56(2):213–20.
55. Haning R, Strawn E, Nolten W. Pathophysiology of the ovarian hyperstimulation syndrome. Obstet Gynecol. 1985;66(2):220–4.
56. Engmann L, Benadiva C, Humaidan P. GnRH agonist trigger for the induction of oocyte maturation in GnRH antagonist IVF cycles: a SWOT analysis. Reprod Biomed Online. 2016;32(3):274–85.
57. Strickland S, Beers W. Studies on the role of plasminogen activa- tor in ovulation. In vitro response of granulosa cells to gonadotro- pins, cyclic nucleotides, and prostaglandins. J Biol Chem. 1976;251(18):5694–702.
58. Eppig JJ. Gonadotropin stimulation of the expansion of cumulus oophori isolated from mice: general conditions for expansion in vitro. J Exp Zool. 1979;208(1):111–20.
59. Zelinski-Wooten M, Hutchison J, Hess D, Wolf D, Stouffer R. Follicle stimulating hormone alone supports follicle growth and oocyte development in gonadotrophin-releasing hormone antagonist-treated monkeys. Hum Reprod. 1995;10(7):1658–66.
60. Yding Andersen C. Effect of FSH and its different isoforms on maturation of oocytes from pre-ovulatory follicles. Reprod Biomed Online. 2002;5(3):232–9.
61. Gonen Y, Balakier H, Powell W, Casper R. Use of gonadotropin releasing hormone agonist to trigger follicular maturation for in vitro fertilization. J Clin Endocrinol Metab. 1990;71(4):918–22.
62. Humaidan P, Papanikolaou E, Tarlatzis B. GnRHa to trigger final oocyte maturation: a time to reconsider. Hum Reprod. 2009;24(10):2389–94.
63. Garcia-Velasco JA, Motta L, Lopez A, Mayoral M, Cerrillo M, Pacheco A. Low-dose human chorionic gonadotropin versus estradiol/progesterone luteal phase support in gonadotropin releasing hormone agonist-triggered assisted reproductive technique cycles: understanding a new approach. Fertil Steril. 2010;94:2820–3.
64. Bodri D, Guillen JJ, Galindo A, Mataro D, Pujol A, Coll O. Triggering with human chorionic gonadotropin or a gonadotropin-releasing hormone agonist in gonadotropin-releasing hormone antagonist-treated oocyte donor cycles: findings of a large retrospective cohort study. Fertil Steril. 2009;91:365–71.
65. Santos-Ribeiro S, Polyzos NP, Stouffs K, De Vos M, Seneca S, Tournaye H, Blockeel C. Ovarian hyperstimulation syndrome after gonadotropin-releasing hormone agonist triggering and "freeze-all": in-depth analysis of genetic predisposition. J Assist Reprod Genet. 2015;32(7):1063–8.
66. Acevedo B, Gomez-Palomares JL, Ricciarelli E, Hernandez ER. Triggering ovulation with gonadotropin-releasing hormone agonists does not compromise embryo implantation rates. Fertil Steril. 2006;86:1682–7.
67. Shapiro BS, Daneshmand ST, Garner FC, Aguirre M, Ross R. Comparison of human chorionic gonadotropin and gonadotropin-releasing hormone agonist for final oocyte maturation in oocyte donor cycles. Fertil Steril. 2007;88:237–9.
68. Galindo A, Bodri D, Guillen JJ, Colodron M, Vernaeve V, Coll O. Triggering with HCG or GnRH agonist in GnRH antagonist treated oocyte donation cycles: a randomised clinical trial. Gynecol Endocrinol. 2009;25:60–6.
69. Hernandez ER, Gomez-Palomares JL, Ricciarelli E. No room for cancellation, coasting, or ovarian hyperstimulation syndrome in oocyte donation cycles. Fertil Steril. 2009;91:1358–61.

70. Engmann L, DiLuigi A, Schmidt D, Nulsen J, Maier D, Benadiva C. The use of gonadotropin-releasing hormone (GnRH) agonist to induce oocyte maturation after cotreatment with GnRH antagonist in high-risk patients undergoing in vitro fertilization prevents the risk of ovarian hyperstimulation syndrome: a prospective randomized controlled study. Fertil Steril. 2008;89:84–91.
71. Frydman R, Parneix I, Belaisch-Allart J, Forman R, Hazout A, Fernandez H, Testart J. LHRH agonists in IVF: different methods of utilization and comparison with previous ovulation stimulation treatments. Hum Reprod. 1988;3(4):559–61.
72. Fanchin R, Peltier E, Frydman R, de Ziegler D. Human chorionic gonadotropin: does it affect human endometrial morphology in vivo? Semin Reprod Med. 2001;19(1):31–5.
73. Papanikolaou EG, Verpoest W, Fatemi H, Tarlatzis B, Devroey P, Tournaye H. A novel method of luteal supplementation with recombinant luteinizing hormone when a gonadotropin-releasing hormone agonist is used instead of human chorionic gonadotropin for ovulation triggering: a randomized prospective proof of concept study. Fertil Steril. 2011;95(3):1174–7.
74. Vloeberghs V, Peeraer K, Pexsters A, D'Hooghe T. Ovarian hyperstimulation syndrome and complications of ART. Best Pract Res Clin Obstet Gynaecol. 2009;23:691–709.
75. Ling LP, Phoon JWL, Lau MSK, Chan JKY, Viardot-Foucault V, Tan TY, Nadarajah S, Tan HH. GnRH agonist trigger and ovarian hyperstimulation syndrome: relook at 'freeze-all strategy'. Reprod Biomed Online. 2014;29:392–4.
76. Gurbuz AS, Gode F, Ozcimen N, Isik AZ. Gonadotrophin-releasing hormone agonist trigger and freeze-all strategy does not prevent severe ovarian hyperstimulation syndrome: a report of three cases. Reprod Biomed Online. 2014;29:541–4.
77. Fatemi HM, Popovic-Todorovic B, Humaidan P, Kol S, Banker M, Devroey P, Garcia-Velasco JA. Severe ovarian hyperstimulation syndrome after gonadotropin-releasing hormone (GnRH) agonist trigger and 'freeze-all' approach in GnRH antagonist protocol. Fertil Steril. 2014;101:1008–11.
78. Maxwell KN, Cholst IN, Rosenwaks Z. The incidence of both serious and minor complications in young women undergoing oocyte donation. Fertil Steril. 2008;90(6):2165–71.
79. Gordon JD, Hopkins KL, Jeffrey RB, Giudice LC. Adnexal torsion: color Doppler diagnosis and laparoscopic treatment. Fertil Steril. 1994;61:383–5.
80. Meyer L, Murphy LA, Gumer A, Reichman DE, Rosenwaks Z, Cholst IN. Risk factors for a suboptimal response to gonadotropin-releasing hormone agonist trigger during in vitro fertilization cycles. Fertil Steril. 2015;104(3):637–42.
81. Kolibianakis E, Albano C, Camus M, Tournaye H, Van Steirteghem A, Devroey P. Prolongation of the follicular phase in *in vitro* fertilization results in a lower ongoing pregnancy rate in cycles stimulated with recombinant follicle-stimulating hormone and gonadotropin-releasing hormone antagonists. Fertil Steril. 2004;82(1):102–7.
82. Melo MA, Meseguer M, Garrido N, Bosch E, Pellicer A, Remohí J. The significance of premature luteinization in an oocyte-donation programme. Hum Reprod. 2006;21(6):1503–7.
83. Bennett SJ, Waterstone JJ, Cheng WC, Parsons J. Complications of transvaginal ultrasound-directed follicle aspiration: a review of 2670 consecutive procedures. J Assist Reprod Genet. 1993;10:72–7.
84. Ludwig AK, Glawatz M, Griesinger G, et al. Perioperative and post-operative complications of transvaginal ultrasound-guided oocyte retrieval: prospective study of >1000 oocyte retrievals. Hum Reprod. 2006;21:3235–40.
85. Dicker D, Ashkenazi J, Feldberg D, et al. Severe abdominal complications after transvaginal ultrasonographically guided retrieval of oocytes for in vitro fertilization and embryo transfer. Fertil Steril. 1993;59:1313–5.
86. Tureck RW, Garcia CR, Blasco L, Mastroianni L Jr. Perioperative complications arising after transvaginal oocyte retrieval. Obstet Gynecol. 1993;81:590–3.
87. Govaerts I, Devreker F, Delbaere A, et al. Short-term medical complications of 1500 oocyte retrievals for in vitro fertilization and embryo transfer. Eur J Obstet Gynecol Reprod Biol. 1998;77:239–43.

88. Roest J, Mous HV, Zeilmaker GH, Verhoeff A. The incidence of major clinical complications in a Dutch transport IVF programme. Hum Reprod Update. 1996;2:345–53.
89. Moini A, Riazi K, Amid V, et al. Endometriosis may contribute to oocyte retrieval-induced pelvic inflammatory disease: report of eight cases. J Assist Reprod Genet. 2005;22:307–9.
90. Bernstein L. Epidemiology of endocrine-related risk factors for breast cancer. J Mammary Gland Biol Neoplasia. 2002;7:3–15.
91. Li LL, Zhou J, Qian XJ, Chen YD. Meta-analysis on the possible association between in vitro fertilisation and cancer risk. Int J Gynecol Cancer. 2013;23:16–24.
92. Siristatidis C, Sergentanis TN, Kanavidis P, Trivella M, Sotiraki M, Mavromatis I, et al. Controlled ovarian hyperstimulation for IVF: impact on ovarian, endometrial and cervical cancer—a systematic review and meta-analysis. Hum Reprod Update. 2013;19:105–23.
93. Kessous R, Davidson E, Meirovitz M, Sergienko R, Sheiner E. The risk of female malignancies after fertility treatments: a cohort study with 25-year follow-up. J Cancer Res Clin Oncol. 2016;142:287–93.
94. Jensen A, Sharif H, Kjaer SK. Use of fertility drugs and risk of uterine cancer: results from a large Danish population-based cohort study. Am J Epidemiol. 2009;170:1408–14.
95. Lerner-Geva L, Liat LG, Rabinovici J, Jaron R, Olmer L, Liraz O, et al. Are infertility treatments a potential risk factor for can- cer development? Perspective of 30 years of follow-up. Gynecol Endocrinol. 2012;28:809–14.
96. Sergentanis TN, Diamantaras AA, Perlepe C, Kanavidis P, Skalki- dou A, Petridou ET. IVF and breast cancer: a systematic review and meta-analysis. Hum Reprod Update. 2014;20:106–23.
97. Lundberg FE, Johansson ALV, Rodriguez-Wallberg K, Brand JS, Czene K, Hall P, Iliadou AN. Association of infertility and fertility treatment with mammographic density in a large screening-based cohort of women: a cross-sectional study. Breast Cancer Res. 2016;18:36.
98. Stoop D, Vercammen L, Polyzos NP, de Vos M, Nekkebroeck J, De Vroey P. Effect of ovarian stimulation and oocyte retrieval on reproductive outcome in oocyte donors. Fertil Steril. 2012;97(6):0015–282.
99. Kramer W, Schneider J, Schultz N. US oocyte donors: a retrospective study of medical and psychologic issues. Hum Reprod. 2009;24:3144–9.
100. Bukulmez O, Li Q, Carr BR, Leander B, Doody KM, Doody KJ. Repetitive oocyte donation does not decrease serum anti-Mullerian hormone level. Fertil Steril. 2010;94:905–12.
101. Kawwass JF, Kissin DM, Kulkarni AD, Creanga AA, Session DR, Callaghan WM, Jamieson DJ. Safety of assisted reproductive technology in the United States, 2000–2011. JAMA. 2015;313(1):88–90.

Chapter 12
Procreative Procrastination: The Ethics of Postponed Parenthood

Daniela Cutas, Anna Smajdor, and Kristien Hens

Introduction

Twelve year old girls "should be taught in school that the 'optimal age' to start a family is in their late twenties" [1]. To expect to be able to postpone reproduction is "to bring cold-hearted calculation into an experience that should result from a burning desire" [2]. "You can't botox your ovaries (…) The problem we have is that women on the outside are shiny, young and youthful and on the inside their ovaries know exactly what it says on their birth certificate" [3]. "Beauty is ageless. Fertility is not" [4]. "Immature men are leaving it too late to have children" [5].

Statements such as these abound in the media and variations of them can be found in medical advice and public health pronouncements [6]. Nevertheless the phenomenon of reproductive postponement appears to be continuing unabated. Across the Western world, the age at which women give birth to their first child has been increasing steadily. In the EU it is now 30.4 [7] (Chap. 2). Similar trends have been reported in the US [8]. This has attracted critical attention, as illustrated in the selection of comments given above. The anxiety surrounding older motherhood is based partly on concerns about increased risks for mothers and

D. Cutas (✉)
Department of Historical, Philosophical and Religious Studies, Umeå University, Umeå, Sweden

Department of Philosophy, Linguistics and Theory of Science, University of Gothenburg, Gothenburg, Sweden
e-mail: daniela.cutas@umu.se

A. Smajdor
Department of Philosophy, Classics, History of Art and Ideas, University of Oslo, Oslo, Norway

K. Hens
Department of Philosophy, University of Antwerp, Antwerp, Belgium

© Springer International Publishing Switzerland 2018

D. Stoop (ed.), *Preventing Age Related Fertility Loss*,
DOI 10.1007/978-3-319-14857-1_12

offspring. Delayed reproduction is riskier than reproduction at the biologically optimal time and health risks involved can affect both mothers and children. Delayed reproduction also carries costs for healthcare providers. These costs relate in part to the greater health needs of older mothers and their offspring, but also to the greater demand for fertility treatments that occurs when people who are ready to have children find they can no longer do so without medical assistance (Chap. 3).

The trend towards later motherhood is commonly attributed to a failure on the part of women to take steps to become parents early in life, leading to later age at first time motherhood, and increased likelihood of fertility problems. Hence, it is believed that this constitutes postponement, or even "procrastination" [2]. However, in this chapter we raise a number of questions about the relationship between increasing age of first time mothers and the factors that give rise to this. Are people (women) *really* procrastinating? And if so, what should be done about it—if anything? We will show that procreative procrastination is best recognized as a symptom of larger and more complex social developments rather than as an isolated phenomenon for which individual women are primarily responsible. The phenomenon of delayed parenthood is taking place in a context of other social, demographic, and medical changes. Because of this, many of the current or suggested strategies for changing women's behaviour are likely to be inadequate.

Do Women Postpone and if So, Why?

Societies in which delayed parenthood is prevalent have adopted various strategies to try to reverse the upward trend in maternal age, and we will discuss some of these in a later section. But the first question to tackle should perhaps be whether women *really are* postponing parenthood, and how it comes about that they increasingly have children at an 'advanced maternal age' rather than earlier in their lives [9]. Our argument here is that some of the negative implications concerning individual choices or failures, which are suggested by terms such as 'postpone' or 'delay' are untenable. If we believe that women are foolishly, ignorantly or lazily making reproductive decisions that harm themselves, their offspring, and society, we might well regard this as amounting to procrastination. However, if young women do not perceive themselves to have the kind of agency required to become parents earlier in life, the negative terms seem less justified. A woman who seeks to become a mother for the first time at 42 *may* have procrastinated. But the mere fact of her being 42 and a first time mother does not in itself justify our concluding this. There are many other factors to take into consideration.

Procrastination, postponement, and delay, are words that are loaded with meaning. Ordinarily, they would imply that the women who seek to reproduce later in life (a) knew from some younger age that they wanted to have children and (b) despite being able to have them earlier, they left it until later. This would be thus the same kind of procrastination/postponement that we can see in people who put off going to the dentist, or making a will. There is no good reason not to do so *now* but they nevertheless delay it. We can contrast this with the example of a person who wants to learn to drive. She knows from a young age that she wants to learn, but cannot do so today because she cannot afford driving lessons. We can imagine another case where someone leaves school and immediately goes into work. As decades pass, he finds himself interested in seeking further education—a wish that he hadn't previously had.

In both of these latter cases, it would seem problematic to suggest that the person had postponed or procrastinated. We might say in the first case, however, that the person *should* have prioritised things differently. Perhaps she should have diverted money towards driving lessons instead of other things. And in the second instance, perhaps we would want to say that the person *should* have considered whether he might at some stage want to go to college, or even that he *should have* had the desire to do so when younger. However, both of these examples show that the questions are complex and normatively loaded. If we think someone should prioritise differently, it suggests that there are competing values at stake. If we don't know what these are, we may have an incomplete view of the picture, and are likely to fail when we tell the person they should choose differently. If we think someone should act on a desire they don't yet have, it suggests that some desires are intrinsically more important than others. As we will go on to show, elements of this kind of value judgement are deeply imbued in the delayed motherhood discourse.

So are young women who do not have children like the people who put off going to the dentist, or more like the other two examples? We will consider the education example first. In this case, the man did not develop the desire to pursue further education until later in life. Similarly, not all women feel sure that they do or will want to have a child while they are young. Some women may think they do, perhaps while they are still children themselves, but might change their view later. Others will find that the wish to become a parent fluctuates or perhaps never materialises at all until they are deemed to be of 'advanced maternal age'. For others, the wish to have a child may depend on many factors (economic stability, career attainment, educational achievement, relationship status, accommodation situation), many of which will be beyond the woman's control. These cases match more closely the example of the woman who cannot afford to learn to drive even though she would like to. In neither case is it clear that postponement or procrastination are appropriate descriptions of what is happening.

Additionally, part of the seriousness of reproductive decisions is their life-changing potential. Because of this, a woman's wish for a child at time X is not in itself a very secure *moral* basis on which to become pregnant. Recognising this, even if a young woman does wish for a child today, but fails to have one, it might not be appropriate to view this as postponement or procrastination. In the paradigmatic examples given above, a person puts off going to the dentist or making a will *for no good reason*. If pressed, they would admit that this is the case. This is precisely the point about delaying, postponing or procrastinating.

In the context of reproduction, the 'no good reason' clause seems harder to substantiate. After all, we are subject to many variable and fluctuating desires; we cannot and should not act on each desire as soon as it emerges. Instead, we have to evaluate and test our desires, including our reproductive aspirations, against our other interests and priorities. This is what our societies and our schools try to emphasise during our formative years. Rather than evidencing irresponsibility, immaturity or lack of information, a reluctance to act immediately on the basis of a desire may on the contrary demonstrate the exercise of our autonomy [10]. That one has to choose between desires may be unfortunate but it may also be ultimately necessary however society is organised.

However, it may still be the case that women are to be criticised for not forming desires that they should have. Reproduction is commonly regarded as a natural aspiration for people in general, especially women. However, in the context of the wider variety of opportunities open to modern women, not all women view reproduction as an inexorable part of their lives. In the past, few women had control over the number or timing of their offspring. They were at the mercy of their own biology and of men. Only in recent decades has this changed for Western women, so that reproduction is no longer a given, but is only one among several possibilities. Moreover, contraception is so strongly normalised in our societies now that an unplanned pregnancy is in itself regarded as a moral failure and a public health problem. It is important here to acknowledge how significant this change is. To the degree that they can effectively control their reproduction, women will not become mothers unless they make a conscious decision to do so.

Making this conscious decision may not be as easy as is popularly thought. The physical, economic and social impact of pregnancy, childbirth, and motherhood, remain formidable. Those who do come to the decision that they want to have children may only reach this point once their most fertile years are over. In view of this, it makes no sense to construe a failure to conceive a child in any particular year as a decision to postpone: "Not deciding to have a child is not logically, morally, or experientially the same as deciding not to have a child" [11].

In short, the language of delay and postponement suggests that women are making conscious, discrete decisions to have children later in life rather than earlier. However, the question, insofar as there is any conscious consideration of it, is not only and always *when* but also *whether*. This challenges the legitimacy of the postponement discourse. It also calls into question the efficacy of many of the strategies that are being proposed to deal with the problem of postponed parenthood—such as educating women to reproduce at a younger age, improving social and working conditions to make things easier for working parents, or using technological solutions such as egg freezing.

Finally, recent surveys of young people indicate their high and increasing vulnerability to economic hardship and difficulties making ends meet in terms of employment, pay, housing, health, wellbeing, confidence, and so on (see e.g. [12]). Youth unemployment rates are higher (in some countries, double) than those of older ages, and women are more vulnerable than men [13]. In these circumstances, it is unrealistic to expect young people to prioritise their reproductive aspirations over other areas of importance in their lives.

In summary, while the trend towards later motherhood is commonly taken to imply postponement, delay or procrastination, the truth is not as simple as this. Women who do wish to have children young are not always able to do so without making considerable sacrifices, e.g. foregoing financial security, or educational advancement, embarking on reproduction without a partner, etc. Women who do not form the wish to have children until they are older also cannot be said to have delayed, postponed or procrastinated, since they could not have known whether the wish to become a mother would in fact develop. Those who argue against postponement therefore would need to think, in the first case, about changing circumstances to allow younger women to reproduce. However, in the second case, it seems that the aim is to *make women want babies while younger.*

Risk

One justification for trying to influence women's reproductive wishes might be to avoid the risks involved in later reproduction. Here, we address the risks of subfertility and the increased medical risks for mothers and children. It is well established that women who wish to become mothers after a certain age are likely to face greater difficulties in realising this desire. With the menopause, natural conception becomes impossible. While men do not face such a dramatic cut-off in their fertility, it is nevertheless the case that older men also face reduced chances of natural conception, and that when both parties are beyond their optimally fertile years, their hopes of parenthood may be thwarted. Treatments such as IVF may help such people overcome age related subfertility. However these treatments in themselves carry medical risks, especially for women, who tend to be the ones to undergo the invasive procedures, even where fertility problems are associated with the male partner. For a woman who does achieve a pregnancy later in life, the risks of conditions such as pre-eclampsia and gestational diabetes [14] are elevated. Delivery for older mothers is also riskier and the likelihood of caesarean section higher. Childbirth takes a toll on mothers of any age, but with existing age related co-morbidities, this is exacerbated.

Although we do not dispute these increased risks it is not clear how or whether they should affect women's reproductive behaviour. Even during women's most fertile years, gestation and childbirth can have significant negative impacts on their health. Women who want to avoid risks related to reproduction would do better to avoid pregnancy altogether. For example, studies suggest that a woman is more likely to die in childbirth than from an abortion [15]. If she avoids pregnancy entirely, she faces neither of these risks [16]. Given that the woman of advanced maternal age is choosing not between earlier motherhood and later motherhood, but between later motherhood and childlessness, the fact that reproduction is riskier than it might have been had she had a child earlier is of limited significance for her decision.

Risks to children, however, might be regarded as being more significant. A woman may accept certain risks for herself, but what about her moral responsibility for deciding to inflict these choices on her child? It has been established that after the age of 35, the quality of a woman's oocytes decreases and that children of older mothers are more likely to be born with conditions such as Down syndrome [18]. It has also been suggested that children born apparently healthy to older mothers are more likely to develop a number of health conditions including childhood cancer [19].

However, difficulties arise in attempting to move from the acknowledgement of such risks, to the conclusion that they should be avoided by preventing the birth of children with these conditions. The potential child of an older mother cannot be benefited by preventing her mother from conceiving her. Nor is it possible to argue that the child is harmed by being brought into existence [20]. Even if, all things considered, it might have been better if the woman had had a child earlier in life, that potential child of the younger woman does not, and never will exist. Aside from this, there are many other complexities related to this question of harm to offspring. For example, studies suggest that IVF itself is associated with increased medical risks for offspring—regardless of parental age [21, 22]. According to a recent study, children born with the help of fertility treatments are at a higher risk of birth defects [23]. Therefore, it might seem that if risk to offspring is the primary concern, rather than worrying about maternal age in particular, we should be arguing against the use of fertility treatments in general.

How About the Men?

When it comes to reproduction, women are still the main focus of attention of policy makers and fertility specialists alike although, as some studies suggest, 40–50% of fertility problems in couples can be attributed to male factors [24]. This seems to operate on a number of different levels. When reproducing at a later age, women are often considered selfish [25, 26]. Fathers, even well in their sixties, are far less confronted with such critiques [11]. Furthermore, men feature highly amongst reasons why women "postpone" parenthood. The strong expectation that parenthood should be pursued as a couple, together with the difficulty of finding a partner with whom to parent, as well as men's own "postponement", are the main reasons invoked by some women as important factors in feeling ready to become a parent [27]. These findings are supported by a host of earlier studies [28]. Such accounts challenge the "career woman" stereotype whilst at the same time drawing attention to the importance of men's role in women's "postponement".

It is often stated that a woman well in her forties may be unable to deal with the broken nights a new-born baby brings, at least far less able than a younger woman [29]. Yet few people raise these objections about men in their forties becoming fathers. The focus on women may suggest that women, more than men, are in need of protection against certain choices, both medically and regarding the ability to put up with broken nights and the general burdens of child rearing. It may suggest that they are too emotionally involved in wanting to have children, and this may cloud their sound judgement regarding what is best for themselves and any children they may have.

This suggests a paternalistic outlook as well as one that tends to further entrench assumptions about women as the sole or primary carer for offspring. However, a part of the context of later childbearing is the fact that relationship expectations have changed in the last decades, as have standards of gender equality and financial independence. Increasingly throughout the Western world, fathers are expected and expect to be active parents, sharing in the care of their children [30]. This is likely to contribute to men becoming more interested in the timing and circumstances in which they become parents.

While there is a marked emphasis on risks to women and risks transmitted by women to offspring, the role of men is seldom discussed in the media and in the literature. This might be taken to suggest that it is only the mother's age that is potentially damaging to offspring. The fact that chromosomal abnormalities such as trisomy-21 are more common in offspring of older mothers has led to the development of prenatal testing techniques such as chorionic villus sampling, amniocentesis and non-invasive prenatal testing (NIPT). For some time the granularity of genomic techniques has only allowed for the detection of abnormalities at the level of the chromosomes. But now that these techniques allow for much more fine-grained screening, it is becoming increasingly evident that paternal age also has an impact on the health of future offspring as well as on fertility.

An over-emphasis on women's roles and responsibilities with regard to reproduction is unfair to both men and women as it obfuscates the fact that sperm is still needed to reproduce, and that male fertility declines with age as well. As we will see in the next section, it has been suggested that *girls* should be educated to think about age-related fertility decline and to plan their reproductive futures. This however may be just as important for men, for whom this uncomfortable truth may hit even harder when they do feel they are mature enough to procreate: many men experience stigma and taboo surrounding their own infertility [31].

Aside from the risks of reduced fertility through paternal age, it has been known for some time that the sperm of older fathers is more likely to contain genetic mutations such as those that cause achondroplasia or Apert syndrome [32, 33]. More recently, it has emerged that epigenetic changes in primordial germ cells that accumulate over a man's lifetime may be passed over to the sperm, and may contribute to the development of conditions such as asthma [34, 35]. The Svanes study found that paternal smoking, even long before conception, affects the likelihood that a child will develop asthma. Interestingly, they did not find a similar effect in women who smoked before conception [35]. The interplay between paternal and maternal factors is as of yet poorly understood [34]. How this information should be dealt with or communicated to potential future parents is yet to be determined, but an approach that points solely to the woman as the main locus of responsibility is inadequate and insufficient.

There is also a broader question here about the direction of research. As we have seen, it is only recently that paternal influences have come to be recognized. Can it be that in the race to identify, measure and control maternal risks, we have failed adequately to make ourselves aware of those pertaining to fathers? If so, this is one instance of the way in which normatively loaded assumptions about gender and responsibility actually determine the path of scientific discovery. This can have the effect of becoming a self-fulfilling prophecy. If we only look for maternal risk, we acquire less evidence for the effect of paternal age on offspring. It is vital to bear this in mind when investigating further aspects of reproductive ageing so as to redress the distorted picture that otherwise emerges.

Education

In the media as well as in the literature it has been pointed out that young women and men are often unaware of the extent to which postponing reproduction may decrease their chance of becoming parents at all. They tend to overestimate their likelihood of successful reproduction as well as likely outcomes of IVF treatments [36, 37]. In this context, it has been suggested that sex education classes in schools should broaden their focus beyond preventing teenage pregnancy and sexually transmitted diseases, to encourage school girls to reflect on their reproductive aspirations when they are still young [38]. A leading UK fertility expert has been quoted as urging that girls as young as 9 years old should be learning about the risks of reproductive postponement [39]. The aim here seems to be that these girls will prioritise reproduction at younger ages as a result of these classes.

Clearly, being informed about one's reproductive potential is a good thing. However, the idea of focusing educational strategies on young girls raises many additional questions: is it feasible to expect a girl of 9 or 15 or 17 to make sense of these messages, while she remains uncertain about so many other aspects of her future life, such as her relationship status or employment? To urge girls to think about their reproductive aspirations at the same time as they are being (in many Western societies) sternly advised to avoid teenage pregnancy at all costs is to send conflicting messages. At best, it seems that these information strategies could be confusing for those they are aimed at. At worst, it might appear that their reproductive lives are subject to ever increasing attention, control, and censure. Aside from these questions, there are problems related to the fact that it is *girls* who are most often the target of the early reproduction messages. Babies are made by men as well as women, yet women are treated as though they are the sole reproductive decision-makers, and are held solely responsible for the demographic shifts in reproductive age.

As we noted above, men also have a role to play in the drift towards later reproduction. It is not as though, while mothers have grown older, fathers have stayed young. Ageing fathers are also at risk of subfertility and their offspring are also at increased risk of medical conditions. Given this, it seems odd, and perhaps unjust, to tell young girls to reproduce earlier (though not too early), without saying anything at all to their male classmates. Boys also need to understand why earlier reproduction might be a good thing for themselves, their partners, their offspring, or for society more generally.

Educational campaigns aimed at young adults are not necessarily a simple solution either. A recent campaign initiated by the Italian government included posters warning young women that it is easier to preserve their beauty than their fertility and pointing out that young people can best be creative by becoming parents and that fertility is a common good. These messages have been met with significant opprobrium both in Italy and internationally [40]. An aggravating factor in this campaign was its failure to acknowledge and address the reasons why parenthood is frequently postponed or avoided altogether in Italy, and which include economic hardships and high unemployment rates. Clearly, whatever measures are taken to reverse the trend of later parenthood and declining fertility rates, they have to be balanced against other socio-economic forces that sustain this trend.

A further important point to mention here with regard to education is that unless policy makers understand the values that people hold, their efforts to change reproductive decision-making are unlikely to succeed. A good example of this is shown in the case of single embryo transfer. A study published in 2007 noted that "women waiting for IVF treatment would prefer to give birth to a child with a chronic disability than never give birth at all" [41]. This study was published at the time when women and fertility clinics were being urged to accept single-embryo-transfer, in order to avoid the risks associated with multiple pregnancies. It was widely assumed that patients continued to accept multiple embryo transfer simply in ignorance of the elevated risks. However, it became increasingly evident that this was not the case. When prospective patients were educated about the risks, they continued to welcome the possibility of multiple pregnancy. For them, the value of a pregnancy, even a medically complicated one; of a baby, even one with a disability, outweighed the greater risk of failing to achieve a pregnancy at all.

There are many parallels between the single embryo transfer debate and the 'postponement' debate. In both cases, there was an assumption that people's behaviour is based simply on lack of information, and a corresponding assumption that the avoidance of medical risk is the sole or primary concern that motivates or should motivate people in their reproductive choices. However, as Scotland et al. observe, even if policy-makers take certain outcomes to be intrinsically bad, unless the people whose behaviour is expected to change *also share this value*, educational campaigns are doomed to failure [41].

In sum, while greater knowledge about one's fertility is a worthy goal, it is unlikely that education is the solution to postponed motherhood. In some respects, it would be strange if this turned out to be the case given that higher educational status is a significant factor associated with postponement [42–44]. That is, the more years of education one has, the fewer children one has, and the later in life one has them. This has implications for the way in which the problem of reproductive postponement is tackled. If we regard postponement as a poor decision resulting from ignorance, it seems paradoxical that it is the most educated women in our societies who are making the most ignorant reproductive decisions.

Technological Solutions

If education—whether of young children or adults, men or women—is unlikely to change the upward trend in reproductive age, another possibility is to accept the phenomenon, and use our medical and technological skills to mitigate the decline in fertility levels. States that are concerned about low fertility may have a reason to consider funding technologies that would allow for a more flexible approach to reproduction. Standard IVF can help with some age-related subfertility problems; however for patients who no longer have viable gametes, this may not enable them to have offspring genetically related to themselves.

Another possibility would be to encourage people to take fertility preservation measures while they are still young enough to produce healthy gametes. Stoop et al. have characterized oocyte banking as a 'preventive intervention' [45]. Viewed in this way, one could argue that states and healthcare providers have good reason to facilitate such techniques as a matter of public health policy. Where such preventive measures have been undertaken, the chances of a successful pregnancy may be significantly increased. Data shows that it is the age of the *egg* rather than the gestational uterus that adversely impacts success rates for IVF [46, 47]. In one sense, then, the risk of subfertility or infertility is a contingent one. There is no absolute cut-off point beyond which a woman cannot carry a pregnancy. If they can obtain 'young' oocytes (whether their own or from a donor), the fact that they are of 'advanced maternal age' need not prevent women from becoming mothers. (In Chap. 13, Mertes discusses in depth the ethics of oocyte freezing.)

While the discourse of 'social freezing' has dominated the media in recent years, it is equally plausible that sperm could and should be pre-emptively frozen. Ovarian or testicular tissue likewise could be preserved for later use. These techniques, apart from offering future options for people who do not currently feel able to reproduce, can circumvent some of the risks involved in using ageing gametes, if the procedure is undertaken while the potential parent is still young.

However, if states or healthcare providers (or employers as in the case of Facebook and Apple) provide gamete freezing for employees, this seems to *encourage* postponement of reproduction. This runs counter to the education and medical exhortations that aim to persuade people (especially women) *not* to postpone. It seems that any concerted strategy carries with it some implicit normative weighting. Currently, women are receiving the message that it is *not* wise to postpone. Yet many do so nevertheless. If gamete freezing becomes more widely accepted, likewise we have an underlying normative message that postponement is acceptable or even commendable. How should we evaluate the impact that this might have on women who prefer to have their children while young? Would they feel pressure to freeze their eggs, and to postpone reproduction against their own inclinations?

There is not scope here to dig very deeply into the ethics of coercion generally. However, it is important to note that women are already subjected to a variety of explicitly and implicitly normative messages *against* postponement. Therefore, if there is an ethical problem involved in attempting to manipulate women's reproductive decisions, simply opting to discourage postponement is not a solution to the problem. The normative loading is there in either case.

Does Later Reproduction Have Any Benefits?

We have focussed so far on the problems associated with delayed parenthood. However, there may also be advantages that need to be considered too. People do not reproduce just to create babies in the best of ways, but to fulfil their ideas about what makes life meaningful [48]. Thus, the timing of reproduction is likely to be affected by other elements in parents' perception of a meaningful life. A specific aspect of older mothers' discourse is the concept of 'being ready' [49]. This feeling of readiness is contingent not on uniquely biological or medical concerns, but on a variety of psychological, social and economic factors, which may include education, employment and feeling mature enough to become a parent.

Becoming a mother between the ages of 30 and 39 has been found to result in better cognitive and behavioural scores for children than doing so at age 23–29 [50, 51]. Women who have children after the age of 35 are statistically more likely to be well educated and to be in employment ([52]: 109). They are more likely than younger mothers to access prenatal care early in their pregnancy, to pursue a healthy lifestyle [53], to breastfeed, and less likely to smoke during the perinatal period [54].

Some women and men who became parents after the age of 40 list "careers with financial security and career-time flexibility, enhanced emotional preparedness, committed co-parenting relationships and a positive overall family experience" as advantages of having delayed childbearing [55]. Another study found that children of women aged 40 had a lower risk of unintentional injuries as well as better language development scores than those of women aged 20 [56]. Children of older parents are less likely to be subjected to harsh or aggressive parental discipline, and have fewer behavioural problems [57].

It has also been suggested that having children after 40 may be positively associated with long-term offspring outcomes, and this macro-level trend may outweigh individual-level risks of postponing. According to one study, "in a regime characterized by improving social conditions, postponing parenthood is beneficial for children even when the individual maternal ageing-related effects might be negative" ([58]: 73). These benefits include an increased likelihood to complete higher education and to perform better in school.

Thus, "postponement" may bring both medical and non-medical benefits not only for parents, but also for children and society at large. "Postponed" parenthood is therefore not straightforwardly a problem, and focusing on its disadvantages only—especially the medical disadvantages—risks brushing over its benefits. Moreover, it may be that in some respects delayed reproduction is a logical corollary of other aspects of our lives, such as the increasing length of childhood, and the high value we ascribe to education. As our lifespans increase, the stretch of time during which we regard ourselves as being young likewise extends. At some stage we have to ask ourselves whether we want our children to become parents while they are still learning how to be adults themselves.

Neoteny

The phenomenon of extended childhood merits further attention in this context as it may help to shed some light on how we should respond to the mismatch between biological and psycho-social imperatives in our reproductive lives. In some species, adults retain juvenile features. For example, dogs are considered neotenic, as they retain playful behaviour throughout their adult life. Humans are also considered a neotenic species, as they retain juvenile features such as a relatively large head in comparison with the rest of their body, a characteristic that is typical for juvenile mammals.

Although human neoteny is often conceived as the retention of (external) juvenile characteristics, the idea could perhaps also be used to illustrate the tendency that our reproductive system is more and more out of tune with our psychological readiness to start a family. Girls in the Western world experience menarche earlier than was the case 150 years ago [59]. At the same time, life expectancy has increased dramatically in the last decades, and women tend to live longer than men. A woman living in France who has a child at 40 can realistically expect to live for another 45 years [60]. Moreover, the age at which biological fertility in both men and women is at its peak may be out of tune with the psychological feeling of being mature enough or ready to become a parent, as well as with the best timing from a social and economic perspective. It may be that it is our own biology that is inconvenient, rather than the rest of our life course [55].

Even if external factors such as the length of education and job insecurity early in life are corrected for, it is possible that this feeling of being not-yet-ready will remain. If so many people only feel mature enough to raise children well past the biologically most optimal time, and if our reproductive system is becoming more and more atavistic, this has far reaching consequences for how we conceive of the distinction between social and medical reasons for preserving fertility. In some cases, technological solutions may be the most realistic option to correct for this conflict: and thus what has been called "social" reasons for preserving fertility may increasingly become one of the indications for mitigating the costs of this mismatch.

Conclusion

The idea that women postpone reproduction has gained some traction in recent years. In this chapter we showed that this perspective omits important parts of the picture. A focus on women's role in reproduction and its postponement neglects the important male factor contributing to infertility and to health risks in offspring. It also denies men the opportunity to discuss their fears regarding their own reproductive potential. Furthermore, it tends to brush over important social and economic factors that also contribute to "postponement". A focus on the risks to both the pregnant woman and her offspring neglects the fact that reproducing at a later age may have benefits as well. Solutions to the problems associated with later parenthood might include a combination of awareness raising (education), technological assistance (such as gamete freezing), and social policies making it easier for people who wish to become parents to do so even at younger ages. A focus solely on medical risks of postponed parenthood can only give a truncated image of the phenomenon, its causes and possible remedies. It suggests that postponement is an individual decision pertaining to the prospective parent (in particular mother), and which can be corrected by informing her of its risks. This is an inaccurate representation of a complex dynamic.

As others have pointed out, there may be no right time to reproduce. Biologically optimal age is but one in a web of forces and contexts which may pull in different directions. We have briefly reviewed some of these in this chapter. We have also pointed out some problems with framing current trends of later reproduction in terms of postponement and with aiming strategies primarily or solely at girls and women.

Key Messages

1. Women tend to be singled out as uninformed postponers responsible for their own difficulty in becoming mothers beyond their most biologically fertile years.
2. Framing later reproduction as "postponement" misrepresents or at least over simplifies the phenomenon of later reproduction.
3. The "postponement" discourse is focused on medical risks and fails to balance these against other risks (such as those arising from the use of fertility treatments themselves) and against possible benefits of later reproduction.
4. For a solution to be effective, it needs to be based on comprehensive understanding of the reasons behind the phenomenon.
5. To some extent, "postponement" may be the result of an atavistic reproductive system that cannot keep up with societal and economic changes: even with the best policies and educational tools in place, the wish to once again reduce the distance between the age of peak biological fertility and readiness to become a parent may be not only misdirected but also futile.

References

1. Teach girls of 12 to start a family by their late 20s. Mail Online. 2016. http://dailymail.co.uk/news/article-3643954/Teach-girls-12-start-family-late-20s-Doctor-s-plea-fears-career-women-risk-missing-motherhood.html.
2. Goring R. The cold-hearted calculation when women choose to freeze their eggs. Herald Scotland. 2016. http://heraldscotland.com/opinion/14554697.display/.
3. You can't fool your ovaries, doctors tell the over-40s. 2016. thetimes.co.uk/article/you-cant-fool-your-ovaries-experts-warn-the-over-40s-hcb5xvfwr.
4. Doctors warn of risks to older mothers. The Guardian. 2009. http://theguardian.com/society/2009/jun/15/older-mothers-health-risks.
5. "Immature" men are leaving it too late to have children. Mail Online. 2016. http://dailymail.co.uk/~/article-3828028/index.html.
6. Mills M, Rindfuss RR, McDonald P, Te Velde E. Why do people postpone parenthood? Reasons and social policy incentives. Hum Reprod Update. 2011;17(6):848–60.
7. Eurostat. Fertility statistics. 2016. http://ec.europa.eu/eurostat/statistics-explained/index.php/Fertility_statistics.
8. Matthews TJ, Hamilton B, Mean age is on the rise: United States, 2000–2014. NCHS Data Brief. 2016; 232.
9. Bernstein S, Wiesemann C. Should postponing motherhood via "social freezing" be legally banned? An ethical analysis. Laws. 2014;3(2):282–300.
10. Bortolotti L, Cutas D. Reproductive and parental autonomy: an argument for compulsory parental education. Reprod Biomed Online. 2009;19(1):5–14.
11. Smajdor A. The ethics of egg donation in the over fifties. Menopause Int. 2008;14(4):173–7.
12. Young women's trust. 2016 annual survey: no country for young women. 2016. http://youngwomenstrust.org/assets/0000/4258/No_country_for_young_women__final_report.pdf.
13. Eurostat. Unemployment statistics. 2016. http://ec.europa.eu/eurostat/statistics-explained/index.php/Unemployment_statistics.
14. Boyd P, DeVigan C, Khoshnood B, Loane M, Garne E, Dolk H. Survey of prenatal screening policies in Europe for structural malformations and chromosome anomalies, and their impact on detection and termination rates for neural tube defects and Down's syndrome. BJOG. 2008;115(6):689–96.
15. Raymond EG, Grimes DA. The comparative safety of legal induced abortion and childbirth in the United States. J Obstet Gynecol. 2012;119(2 Pt 1):215–9.
16. Smajdor A. In defense of ectogenesis. Camb Q Healthc Ethics. 2012;21(1):90–103.
17. Broekmans FJ, Knauff EAH, te Velde ER, Macklon NS, Fauser BC. Female reproductive ageing: current knowledge and future trends. Trends Endocrinol Metab. 2007;18(2):58–65.
18. Snijders RJM, Sundberg K, Holzgreve W, Henry G, Nicolaides KH. Maternal age- and gestation-specific risk for trisomy 21. Ultrasound Obstet Gynecol. 1999;13(3):167–70.
19. Johnson KJ, Carozza SE, Chow EJ, Fox EE, Horel S, McLaughlin CC, et al. Parental age and risk of childhood cancer: a pooled analysis. Epidemiology. 2009;20(4):475–83.
20. Smajdor A. How useful is the concept of the "harm threshold" in reproductive ethics and law? Theor Med Bioeth. 2014;35(5):321–36.
21. Hart R, Norman RJ. The longer-term health outcomes for children born as a result of IVF treatment. Part II--Mental health and development outcomes. Hum Reprod Update. 2013;19(3):244–50.
22. Lazaraviciute G, Kauser M, Bhattacharya S, Haggarty P, Bhattacharya S. A systematic review and meta-analysis of DNA methylation levels and imprinting disorders in children conceived by IVF/ICSI compared with children conceived spontaneously. Hum Reprod Update. 2014;20(6):840–52.
23. Davies MJ, Moore VM, Willson KJ, Van Essen P, Priest K, Scott H, et al. Reproductive technologies and the risk of birth defects. N Engl J Med. 2012;366(19):1803–13.

24. Kumar N, Singh AK. Trends of male factor infertility, an important cause of infertility: a review of literature. J Hum Reprod Sci. 2015;8(4):191–6.
25. Cutas D. Postmenopausal motherhood: immoral, illegal? A case study. Bioethics. 2007;21(8):458–63.
26. Shaw RL, Giles DC. Motherhood on ice? A media framing analysis of older mothers in the UK news. Psychol Health. 2009;24(2):221–36.
27. Baldwin K, Culley L, Hudson N, Mitchell H. Oocyte cryopreservation for social reasons: demographic profile and disposal intentions of UK users. Reprod Biomed Online. 2015;31(2):239–45.
28. Balbo N, Billari F, Mills M. Fertility in advanced societies: a review of research. Eur J Popul. 2013;29(1):1–38.
29. Cutas D, Smajdor A. Postmenopausal motherhood reloaded: advanced age and in vitro derived gametes. Hypatia. 2015;30(2):386–402.
30. Collier R, Sheldon S. Fragmenting fatherhood. A socio-legal study. Oxford: Hart Publishing 2008.
31. Wischmann T, Thorn P. (Male) infertility: what does it mean to men? New evidence from quantitative and qualitative studies. Reprod Biomed Online. 2013;27(3):236–43.
32. Glaser RL, Broman KW, Schulman RL, Eskenazi B, Wyrobek AJ, Jabs EW. The paternal-age effect in Apert syndrome is due, in part, to the increased frequency of mutations in sperm. Am J Hum Genet. 2003;73(4):939–47.
33. Wyrobek AJ, Eskenazi B, Young S, Arnheim N, Tiemann-Boege I, Jabs EW, et al. Advancing age has differential effects on DNA damage, chromatin integrity, gene mutations, and aneuploidies in sperm. Proc Natl Acad Sci. 2006;103(25):9601–6.
34. Day J, Savani S, Krempley BD, Nguyen M, Kitlinska JB. Influence of paternal preconception exposures on their offspring: through epigenetics to phenotype. Am J Stem Cell. 2016;5(1):11–8.
35. Svanes C, Koplin J, Skulstad SM, Johannessen A, Bertelsen RJ, Benediktsdottir B, et al. Father's environment before conception and asthma risk in his children: a multi-generation analysis of the respiratory health in Northern Europe study. Int J Epidemiol. 2016. [online first].
36. Schmidt L. Should men and women be encouraged to start childbearing at a younger age? Expert Review of Obstetrics and Gynecology 2010;5(2):145–7.
37. Lemoine ME, Ravitsky V, Sleepwalking into infertility: The need for a public health approach toward advanced maternal age. Am J Bioeth 2015;15(11):37–46.
38. The doctor warning 15-year-olds about their declining fertility. The Guardian. 2016. http://theguardian.com/education/2016/may/17/the-doctor-warning-15-year-olds-about-their-declining-fertility.
39. Nargund G. Why boys should also receive fertility education in schools. The Huffington Post. 2016. http://huffingtonpost.co.uk/dr-geeta-nargund/why-boys-should-also-rece_b_11258112.html.
40. Italy's fertility day posters aren't just sexist—they're echoes of a fascist past. The Guardian. 2016. http://theguardian.com/commentisfree/2016/sep/05/italys-fertility-day-posters-sexist-echoes-of-fascist-past.
41. Scotland GS, McNamee P, Peddie VL, Bhattacharya S. Safety versus success in elective single embryo transfer: women's preferences for outcomes of in vitro fertilisation. BJOG International. J Obstet Gynaecol. 2007;114(8):977–83.
42. Eriksson C, Larsson M, Skoog Svanberg A, Tydén T. Reflections on fertility and postponed parenthood—interviews with highly educated women and men without children in Sweden. Uppsala J Med Sci. 2013;118(2):122–9.
43. Neels K, Murphy M, Ní Bhrolcháin M, Beaujouan É. Further estimates of the contribution of rising educational participation to fertility postponement: a model-based decomposition for the UK, France and Belgium. In Population Association of America 2014 Annual Meeting, Boston, pp. 1–3; 2014.
44. van Roode T, Sharples K, Dickson N, Paul C. Life-course relationship between socioeconomic circumstances and timing of first birth in a birth cohort. PLoS One. 2017;12(1):e0170170.

45. Stoop D, van der Veen F, Deneyer M, Nekkebroeck J, Tournaye H. Oocyte banking for anticipated gamete exhaustion (AGE) is a preventive intervention, neither social nor nonmedical. Reprod Biomed Online. 2014;28:548–51.
46. Hourvitz A, Machtinger R, Maman E, Baum M, Dor J, Levron J. Assisted reproduction in women over 40 years of age: how old is too old? Reprod Biomed Online. 2009;19:599–603.
47. Navot D, Bergh PA, Williams MA, Garrisi GJ, Guzman I, Sandler B, Grunfeld L. Poor oocyte quality rather than implantation failure as a cause of age-related decline in female fertility. Lancet. 1991;337:1375–7.
48. Dion KK. Delayed parenthood and women's expectations about the transition to parenthood. Int J Behav Dev. 1995;18(2):315–33.
49. Shelton N, Johnson S. "I think motherhood for me was a bit like a double-edged sword": the narratives of older mothers. J Community Appl Soc Psychol. 2006;16(4):316–30.
50. Goisis A, How are children of older mothers doing? Evidence from the United Kingdom. Biodemography and Social Biology 2015;61(3):231–251.
51. Goisis A, Schneider DC, Myrskylä M. The reversing association between advanced maternal age and child cognitive ability: evidence from three UK birth cohorts. Int J Epidemiol 2017. doi:10.1093/ije/dyw354.
52. Graham H. Hardship & Health in women's lives. London: Routledge; 2014.
53. Tough SC, Newburn-Cook C, Johnston DW, Svenson LW, Rose S, Belik J. Delayed childbearing and its impact on population rate changes in lower birth weight, multiple birth, and preterm delivery. Pediatrics. 2002;109(3):399–403.
54. Boivin J, Rice F, Hay D, Harold G, Lewis A, van den Bree M, Thapar A. Associations between maternal older age, family environment and parent and child wellbeing in families using assisted reproductive techniques to conceive. Soc Sci Med. 2009;68(11):1948–55.
55. Mac Dougall K, Beyene Y, Nachtigall RD, 'Inconvenient biology': advantages and disadvantages of first'time parenting after age 40 using in vitro fertilization. Human Reproduction 2012:27(4):1058–65.
56. Sutcliffe A, Barnes J, Belsky J, Gardiner J, Melhuish E. The health and development of children born to older mothers in the United Kingdom: observational study using longitudinal cohort data. BMJ. 2012;345:e5116.
57. Trillingsgaard T, Sommer D. Associations between older maternal age, use of sanctions, and children's socio-emotional development through 7, 11, and 15 years. Eur J Dev Psychol. 2016:1–5.
58. Barclay K, Myrskylä M. Advanced maternal age and offspring outcomes: reproductive aging and counterbalancing period trends. Popul Dev Rev. 2016;42(1):69–94.
59. Pierce M, Hardy R. Commentary: The decreasing age of puberty—as much a psychosocial as biological problem? Int J Epidemiol. 2012;41(1):300–2.
60. Eurostat. Mortality and life expectancy statistics. 2016. http://ec.europa.eu/eurostat/statistics-explained/index.php/Mortality_and_life_expectancy_statistics.

Chapter 13
Ethical Aspects of AGE Banking

Heidi Mertes

Introduction

Although the first healthy live birth from a frozen human egg cell dates back to 1986, egg freezing has long been so inefficient that it was hardly considered a valid treatment option [1]. However, with improvements in both the slow freezing technique and ultra-rapid cooling by vitrification, oocyte cryopreservation (OC) has become an efficient procedure with high survival rates after thawing [2–8].

The primary application of this new technology was to bank eggs for women who are at risk of losing their fertility due to cancer, cancer treatment or other grave illnesses. However, not only cancer patients are at risk of losing their fertility, but all women in their late thirties are. Therefore, also for this group, OC could be beneficial. However, the expansion of the option of OC for 'medical reasons' to OC for 'non-medical reasons', 'social reasons' or 'anticipated gamete exhaustion' (AGE-banking) [9] was not met with the same enthusiasm. In 2007, the American Society for Reproductive Medicine (ASRM) stated that "Oocyte cryopreservation is an experimental procedure that should not be offered or marketed as a means to defer reproductive aging, primarily because data relating to clinical outcomes are limited. [...] However, unlike healthy women, [women with cancer or other illnesses requiring immediate treatments that seriously threaten their future fertility] may have no viable options and therefore may be appropriate candidates for such treatment despite its experimental status" [10]. The European Society for Human Reproduction and Embryology (ESHRE) took a similar stand: "In view of the lack of success and clinical applications in the case of ovarian tissue, this application should not be offered to women as a means to preserve their fertility potential when there is no immediate threat to their fertility. According to similar reasoning, oocyte freezing

H. Mertes
Bioethics Institute Ghent, Ghent University, Blandijnberg 2, 9000 Ghent, Belgium
e-mail: Heidi.Mertes@UGent.be

© Springer International Publishing Switzerland 2018

D. Stoop (ed.), *Preventing Age Related Fertility Loss*,
DOI 10.1007/978-3-319-14857-1_13

for fertility preservation without a medical indication should not be encouraged." [11]. Given the explosion of new research data in the years that followed, several authors have called directly upon ASRM and ESHRE for a less restrictive attitude [12, 13]. This resulted in a revision of the ESHRE-guidelines in 2012, now stating that "[i]n the light of new scientific developments, and after considering relevant ethical arguments [...] oocyte cryopreservation to improve prospects of future child bearing should also be available for non-medical reasons" [14]. The ASRM, however, despite lifting the 'experimental' label from OC for medical purposes in 2012, maintained its stance that OC should not be offered for non-medical reasons due to a lack of data for this specific indication and due to the fact that "[m]arketing this technology for the purpose of deferring childbearing may give women false hope and encourage women to delay childbearing" [15].

In this chapter, the different arguments pro and con OC to counter age-related fertility decline will be presented and critically assessed. This overview will show that although there are no strong arguments against the principle of AGE-banking, the ethical concerns that are voiced in regard to the technology do point at legitimate concerns about the way it is/should be offered to patients. As a preliminary remark, please note that although safety is obviously an important ethical concern for all new medical technology, it will not be discussed in this chapter.

Fundamental Objections Against AGE Banking

The Argument from Nature

A first set of fundamental objections against AGE-banking relate to the idea that this technology pushes the boundaries of nature. The age at which the average woman becomes infertile is then not merely labelled as a biological fact, as the age at which women *can* no longer have children, but rather as the age at which women *should* no longer have children. In ethical theory, this phenomenon is known as the is-ought fallacy. Unless if one starts from the religious belief that everything was created for a clear purpose and that we live in the best of all possible worlds, the (average) natural state of things does not teach us anything about how things ought to be. This also implies that there is no obvious reason why medical interventions should be limited to preserving or restoring the natural state of things—as is done in 'medical' egg freezing—and should not be used to counter natural phenomena that have a negative impact on our wellbeing. It should be remarked that many illnesses are age-related, just as the decline in female fertility, and that many medical interventions are performed to solve inconveniences that may be considered 'normal' if they occur at a certain age. In fact, not much of modern day medicine would remain, if we were to cancel all interventions for age-related health problems. Yet, nobody seems to be opposed to the treatment of Alzheimer's disease or osteoporosis. The distinction between medical and non-medical egg freezing based on the idea that aging is not a medical problem is therefore problematic. If we have good reasons to counteract infertility for women with a desire for parenthood, then it matters little what the cause of the pending infertility is.

Also, besides the fact that the distinction between medical and non-medical OC is irrelevant, it is also a false distinction in the sense that there is a grey area in between these two applications [9]. For instance, should women who request OC due to a prognosis of unexplained premature ovarian insufficiency be regarded as freezing for medical or non-medical reasons? Even for cancer patients, certain regimens of radiation or chemotherapy will lead to immediate sterility in (reproductively speaking) older women, but not in younger women. The reasons for the former to store oocytes are therefore both disease-related and age-related. In this chapter, I will maintain the term 'AGE banking', which allows for a wide interpretation, although many of the objections discussed will be aimed primarily at egg freezing for healthy women.

Medicalization

A related objection against AGE-banking is that it provides a medical solution for a problem that in essence is not a medical problem, but a societal one, namely the steady rise in women's age at first childbirth (now on average between 25 and 35 years old). This can then be attributed either to the woman herself or to the way the labour market is structured.

If women are held accountable for 'delaying' childbearing due to 'lifestyle choices', the non-medical alternative to OC is obvious and simple: women should reproduce earlier. This is however easier said than done. The most important reason for banking eggs in healthy women is the lack of a partner [16–18]. Should we thus encourage women to become single mothers? Should we advise them not to wait for Mr. Right, but go for Mr. Good Enough? Besides the most important factor of finding a suitable partner to share parenthood with, several studies have found that women also find it increasingly important to first complete their education, have financial security and good housing before taking on the responsibility of parenthood [19, 20]. These are not trivial desires, but relevant for the wellbeing of themselves and their future children. Bonneux et al. [21] have therefore argued that the rise in the age at first childbirth is a trend that increases overall wellbeing and that should not be regretted in itself, even if it is regrettable that the peak of natural female fertility does not coincide with the moment at which women would preferably have their children.

Alternatively, rather than holding women accountable for the rising age at first childbirth, society might be blamed, in the sense that many women experience difficulties in starting a parental project during their reproductive lifespan due to professional obligations. While fertility preservation can offer a solution to this problem once it presents itself, it does not tackle the root cause. As mentioned by Goold and Savulescu [22], "one might ask whether we actually help women [...] by taking for granted their bad employment situation and offering them egg freezing to deal with it". Fertility preservation for social reasons is then a type of unnecessary medicalization of society that can be avoided by creating a better social climate for working mothers. However, societal change takes time. While we might attempt to tackle the (hypothetical) root cause of delayed childbearing by making it easier for young parents (both women *and* men) to combine personal and professional responsibilities, this is unfortunately not a solution for women who are in their late thirties and involuntarily childless today. Therefore, long term solutions to the benefit of future generations should not prevent us from offering practical solutions to the present generation [23, 24]. Moreover, keeping in mind that lack of a partner is the primary reason to request AGE banking, we should be sceptical that reforms in the labour market will reduce the demand for AGE banking. At the same time, we should remain vigilant that the option of AGE banking is not invoked as an excuse to invest less in reforms in the labour marked that enable a better combination of professional and parental obligations.

A Negative Impact on Society

Related to the argument that women's employment situation does not allow them to reproduce at a young age, there is a concern that the offer of AGE banking will increase the pressure on women to invest in their careers while they are young at the expense of pursuing parenthood. This concern became especially convincing when Facebook and Apple announced that they would start offering OC to their female employees. As argued elsewhere, even if AGE banking in itself may not be ethically problematic, the offer by employers is [25]. For such a policy to be implemented with respect for women's reproductive autonomy, a substantial number of conditions need to be fulfilled, which can be reduced to three categories: (1) women should understand the benefits, risks and limitations, (2) women should feel no pressure to take up the offer; (3) the offer should have no negative effect on other family-friendly policies and should in fact be accompanied by such policies. Fulfilling these conditions may turn out to be impossible. Thus, regardless of companies' possible good intentions, women's reproductive autonomy is not well served by offering them company-sponsored AGE banking.

Another concern is that the offer of AGE-banking may cause an increase in the average age at which women become mothers. Although this effect is possible, there are various reasons why it is unlikely that this effect would be significant. First, the number of women opting to bank oocytes is likely to remain a small fraction of all women desiring to become mothers, as the procedure requires a substantial physical and financial effort. Second, it is wrong to assume that these women make a choice between reproducing 'now' or reproducing a couple of years later. For many of the women opting for AGE banking, reproducing at the moment of freezing is not an option (due to lack of a partner, as mentioned). The more likely alternatives are thus either not reproducing at all, or reproducing via donor oocytes. Third, women who bank oocytes on average do so in their late thirties and on average consider the maximum age to use the oocytes below 44 years [26]. This means that even for the small fraction of women who would consider a pregnancy at the time of freezing if AGE banking were not available, motherhood is only 'deferred' for about 5 years. In conclusion, the most likely effect of offering fertility preservation to healthy women is not a decline in the number of young mothers but a small incline in the number of older mothers. Whether an increase in the age of mothers is problematic in itself, is discussed in Chap. 12.

Fundamental Arguments for AGE Banking

Gender Equality

An argument in favour of AGE banking is that this intervention is emancipatory in nature as it can fix the factual discrimination between men and women in regard to their reproductive lifespan: if men are able to conceive children at an advanced age, then women should have the same liberty. This is again an example of the is-ought-fallacy. The mere biological fact that a 70-year old man is capable of conceiving children, says nothing about the moral reasons for (not) doing so. However, as reproductive freedom is highly valued in our society, we do not impose forced sterilization on men above a certain age. Reproduction at an advanced age is thus a liberty right, but that does not mean that it is also a claim right. That means that if an infertile senior citizen (male or female) applies for IVF treatment, it may not be granted based on considerations regarding the welfare of the future child. Given the fact that pregnancy complications are an additional concern in the case of women, a lower cut-off age in ART for women than for men may be justified.

Reproductive Autonomy

The main argument for AGE banking is that it increases reproductive autonomy. Due to this new technology, women are theoretically able to extend their reproductive lifespan and are thus less dependent on donor oocytes if they wish to reproduce at an age at which their ovarian reserves are depleted (see below). As mentioned above, the age at which women desire to have children rises and not all women succeed in finding a partner with whom to share parenthood before the decline of their fertility. When single, childless women reach their late thirties and still want to become mothers, they—unlike men—are under pressure to find a partner fast and embark on parenthood with that new partner fast, or resort to single parenthood. AGE banking can relieve women of this pressure by offering them a couple more years to find a suitable partner, thus allowing for more autonomous choices. Caveats are that only a limited number of oocytes can be banked, so that a pregnancy—let alone a live birth—can certainly not be guaranteed and that women still face legal restrictions on the age until which they can use their banked oocytes to (try to) establish a pregnancy.

An absolute prerequisite for AGE banking to positively influence reproductive autonomy is that women receive correct information about the possibilities and limitations. The overly optimistic portrayal of AGE banking as 'insurance against infertility' or as a means to defer childbearing while retaining fertility misguides women about the limitations. If a woman with a very strong desire for parenthood would defer childbearing relying on banked oocytes and subsequently fails to achieve a pregnancy with those banked oocytes, her reproductive autonomy was very ill-served by AGE banking.

Psychological Benefit

Linked to reproductive autonomy and the pressure on finding a suitable partner when a woman approaches the end of her reproductive lifespan is the observation that women may not only derive a clinical benefit (the chance of conceiving a child), but also a psychological benefit from knowing that there is still 'a chance' for her to have children, regardless of whether she ever actually uses her stored eggs. Research by Stoop et al. [26] shows that even women who have banked oocytes but have never used them or no longer envisage using them do not regret their decision to bank and would do so again in similar circumstances. Also, some women decide a couple of years after banking that they will embark on single parenthood although their preferential life plan involved building a family with a partner. Banking then allowed them some extra time to consider the option of single parenthood without Damocles' sword hanging above their heads.

Self-donation

A strong argument for allowing AGE banking is that it is in fact a form of oocyte donation which does not involve a third party [13, 27]. If a woman is currently unable to conceive due to a depletion of her ovarian reserve, she can establish a pregnancy with donor oocytes, but there are some drawbacks to this option. First, the resulting child will not have a genetic connection with the mother. Although this is not necessarily problematic, it is a suboptimal option for many people, either because they identify parenthood with genetic parenthood (or at least presuppose that one is 'more' of a parent when there is a genetic connection) or because they fear a disruption of their family unit if the donor would claim a role or if the child would regard the donor as the 'real' mother [28]. Second, oocyte donation requires that a healthy woman is subjected to ovarian stimulation and oocyte retrieval. These are unpleasant and time-consuming procedures with (limited) risks involved, which hold no benefit for the woman who is subjected to these risks. Both donor anonymity and open identity donation are potentially problematic for the donor, in the former case because she might want to know the person resulting from her donation, in the latter case because she might *not* want to be contacted by that person. As we currently allow donor conception despite these drawbacks, it would be inconsistent not to allow a woman to donate oocytes to her future self. In this case the genetic link is maintained and the person subjected to the risks of ovarian stimulation is the same person as the one who reaps the benefit of (potential) parenthood. The only dissimilarity that might be invoked to justify a different approach is that in the case of 'regular' oocyte donation, the need for a donor oocyte is present, whereas when a woman decides to bank oocytes for future use, she can never be certain that there will ever be an actual need. Therefore, the effort might be in vain.

Concerns About Improper Introduction into the Clinic

Utility

The major problem for AGE banking is that in many cases, it will be a medical intervention without clinical benefit. Few women will mimic the best case scenario—which is the one that commercial companies offering AGE banking are most likely to highlight—in which women between 30 and 35 realise that they will not be in ideal circumstances to reproduce in the coming years, store their oocytes, then meet Mr. Right, build up a stable relationship and come back to the clinic to use their oocytes around age 40 (when their ovarian reserve is depleted), establish a pregnancy and become mothers. If women bank their oocytes at a younger age, the quality of these oocytes—and therefore the chance to achieve a healthy live birth—is better, but then there is a large chance that they will never return to use them, as there is still a big chance that they will be able to reproduce naturally during their reproductive lifespan. If women bank their oocytes at an older age, there is a larger chance that they might need them (in the sense that their window of opportunity for natural reproduction is about to close), but the odds of achieving a live birth are a lot smaller as the quality of the oocytes will be a lot poorer [29]. In practice, it turns out that most 'AGE bankers' correspond more to the latter category. Women do not proactively freeze eggs during their twenties or early thirties in a well thought-out plan of achieving their career goals first and focussing on parenthood later. Instead, women turn to AGE banking as a last resort. This also means that many women present themselves at the clinic at a moment when the intervention can bring little benefit for them because ovarian stimulation may only yield a couple of bad quality oocytes which are unlikely to lead to a viable pregnancy.

Although it is too early to draw any definitive conclusions, preliminary studies indicate that the eventual utility of the procedure may indeed be low. For example, Garcia-Velasco et al. [30] report that from 560 non-oncological patients banking oocytes between 2007 and 2012, only 30 had returned for treatment in 2013 and of those 30 there were 5 live births and 8 on-going pregnancies at the time of publication. In a study by Stoop et al. [26] only half the women who banked oocytes anticipates using them in the future. However, this study also confirms that besides the clinical utility of achieving a live birth, there is also a psychological benefit to consider, as the great majority of women was still positive about the decision to store oocytes, also if they anticipate not using them. In any case, counselling for women who inquire about the possibility of oocyte banking should include information about the possibly low utility of the procedure and thus of their investment.

Information

Not only information about utility needs to be provided to potential oocyte bankers, but also, as previously argued, information about the success rates, stratified by age [29]. Ideally, not the chance of a live birth per oocyte should be given, but the cumulative live birth rate with the number of oocytes that are expected to be banked. This information is however not always available. Cil et al. [31] have constructed a model for the age specific probability of live-birth for different numbers of thawed oocytes (based on a meta-analysis) and report a probability of live-birth for a 38-year old woman (at the time of freezing) of 15% for 6 thawed oocytes (after vitrification). 37–38 has been reported as the average age of women opting for AGE-banking [16, 18, 32–35]. It is clear that for this group, metaphors such as 'putting fertility on ice', 'stopping the reproductive clock', 'fertility insurance' or 'fertility preservation' are misleading, as the chance that they will not be able to conceive with their banked oocytes appears to be larger than the chance that they will succeed.

Also for younger women, the danger of misinformation is lurking. Although there are currently few reports of young women storing oocytes with the explicit purpose of postponing motherhood, some commercial companies are definitely aiming at young women invested in their careers to 'sell' their intervention to, targeting them through events such as egg freezing parties. In this situation, the danger is that women do not realise that postponing parenthood always results in a decline in the chance of establishing a pregnancy, even when eggs are banked, as these banked eggs are always limited in number. A woman may thus enter into AGE banking believing that her desire for children is 'safe', while it is not. According to the model by Cil et al., a 28 year old women would have a 27% live birth rate for 6 thawed oocytes (after vitrification).

Misleading and Coercive Offers

Concerns regarding the clinical utility and the provision of information are both linked to the commercialisation of autologous oocyte banking. When financial profit becomes a factor that influences the offer of oocyte banking or even becomes the goal, the probability that women's attention will be drawn to the drawbacks or that they will be encouraged to reconsider their plans of banking is low. Reference is easily made to reproductive autonomy in this context: if women want to bank their oocytes—even despite the low utility—they should have the liberty to do so and therefore commercial companies should be free to offer it to them. However, respecting an autonomous choice requires that the choice is truly autonomous, that is, that it is based on all the relevant information and free from outside pressure. This is more easily achieved in a non-commercial context.

Besides the fear for misleading offers by commercial egg banking companies, fears exist regarding coercive offers by employers. As discussed above (see section "A Negative Impact on Society"), even if the rationale behind including egg banking in a benefit package would be to increase reproductive autonomy, the chance that the opposite—a decrease in reproductive autonomy—would result is very large.

Access

If employers cannot include egg banking in their healthcare benefit package, then how should egg banking be financed? If the banking woman pays, there are concerns about distributive justice in the sense that this technology will only be available to the segment of society that can afford it. However, allocating public healthcare funds to AGE banking is not straightforward either, given the fact that healthcare funding is limited and should thus be allocated to the most urgent healthcare needs. Also, the limited utility is an argument against incorporating AGE banking in publicly funded healthcare. Cost-efficiency is also a relevant factor to be considered here. However, as argued elsewhere [36], in a system where IVF is reimbursed, it would be inconsistent to cover IVF treatment with donor oocytes for women who are infertile due to aging, but not with their own previously banked oocytes. Thus, in such a context, at least the second part of the procedure, that is thawing, fertilising and transferring any resulting embryos, should be reimbursed. This does not necessarily imply that the first step of the procedure, namely the costs related to ovarian stimulation, oocyte retrieval, oocyte freezing and storage need to be covered, although there are good reasons to argue for full coverage, a cash back-system or more free transfer cycles [36].

Conclusion

Despite the original opposition against AGE banking for healthy women, AGE banking has found its way to the clinic rather fast. One reason for this evolution may be that a number of the initial ethical objections to oocyte freezing for so-called 'social' or 'non-medical' reasons were not very convincing, especially given the contrast with the warm welcome oocyte banking received in the field of oncofertility. The arguments that we should not try to circumvent natural boundaries, solve societal problems with medical solutions or that AGE banking will have a negative impact on society are either flawed or only partially convincing. On the other side of the debate, the argument that we should allow AGE banking to combat gender inequality in terms of the maximal age at childbirth was dismissed, but the argument that women's reproductive autonomy should be respected, that this technology may not only clinically, but also psychologically benefit patients and that it is inconsistent to support egg donation by others, but not autologous egg donation appear to carry some weight.

However, even if there are good arguments to bring AGE banking to the clinic, a cautious approach is warranted. First of all, the utility of the procedure may be low and women may be overly optimistic about their chances of conceiving after AGE banking. They should therefore be properly counselled and sufficiently informed about their personal chances of success. Misleading information by commercial companies and coercive offers from companies to their female employees are to be avoided and finally, reflection is needed on access to the technology and on the extent in which reimbursement by public healthcare is desirable.

Key Message

1. The distinction between oocyte cryopreservation for medical reasons or non-medical/social reasons is ill-founded.
2. In principle, oocyte cryopreservation for healthy women could increase reproductive autonomy and benefit women both clinically and psychologically.
3. The biggest ethical concerns are linked to the implementation in the clinical context.
4. Proper counselling aimed at insuring realistic expectations towards the success rate of the procedure and countering misleading information is a necessary condition that should be guaranteed at all times.
5. Reflection is needed on access to the technology.

References

1. Gook D. History of oocyte cryopreservation. Reprod Biomed Online. 2011;23:281–9.
2. Almodin CG, Minguetti-Camara VC, Paixao CL, Pereira PC. Embryo development and gestation using fresh and vitrified oocytes. Hum Reprod. 2010;25:1192–8.
3. Cobo A, Kuwayama M, Perez S, Ruiz A, Pellicer A, Remohi J. Comparison of concomitant outcome achieved with fresh and cryopreserved donor oocytes vitrified by the Cryotop method. Fertil Steril. 2008;69:1657–64.
4. Grifo JA, Noyes N. Delivery rate using cryopreserved oocytes is comparable to conventional in vitro fertilization using fresh oocytes: potential fertility preservation for female cancer patients. Fertil Steril. 2010;93:391–6.
5. Noyes N, Knopman J, Labella P, McCaffrey C, Clark-Williams M, Grifo J. Oocyte cryopreservation outcomes including pre-cryopreservation and post-thaw meiotic spindle evaluation following slow cooling and vitrification of human oocytes. Fertil Steril. 2010;94:2078–82.
6. Noyes N, Porcu E, Borini A. Over 900 oocyte cryopreservation babies born with no apparent increase in congenital anomalies. Reprod Biomed Online. 2009;18:769–76.

7. Rienzi L, Romano S, Albricci L, Maggiulli R, Capalbo A, Baroni E, et al. Embryo development of fresh 'versus' vitrified metaphase II oocytes after ICSI: a prospective randomized sibling-oocyte study. Hum Reprod. 2010;25:66–73.
8. Trokoudes KM, Pavlides C, Zhang X. Comparison outcome of fresh and vitrified donor oocytes in an egg-sharing donation program. Fertil Steril. 2011;95:1996–2000.
9. Stoop D, van der Veen F, Deneyer M, Nekkebroeck J, Tournaye H. Oocyte banking for anticipated gamete exhaustion (AGE) is a preventive intervention, neither social nor nonmedical. Reprod Biomed Online. 2014;28:548–51.
10. Practice Committee of the SART & ASRM. Essential elements of informed consent for elective oocyte cryopreservation: a Practice Committee opinion. Fertil Steril. 2007;88:1495–6.
11. ESHRE Task Force on Ethics and Law. Taskforce 7: Ethical considerations for the cryopreservation of gametes and reproductive tissues for self use. Hum Reprod. 2004;19:460–2.
12. Homburg R, van der Veen F, Silber SJ. Oocyte vitrification-Women's emancipation set in stone. Fertil Steril. 2009;91:1319–20.
13. Rybak EA, Lieman HJ. Egg freezing, procreative liberty and ICSI: the double standards confronting elective selfdonation of oocytes. Fertil Steril. 2009;92:1509–12.
14. Dondorp W, de Wert G, Pennings G, Shenfield F, Devroey P, Tarlatzis B, et al. Oocyte cryopreservation for age-related fertility loss. Hum Reprod. 2012;27(5):1231–7.
15. ASRM. Mature oocyte cryopreservation: a guideline. Fertil Steril. 2012;99:37–43.
16. Baldwin K, Culley L, Hudson N, Mitchell H, Lavery S. Oocyte cryopresersvation for social reasons: demographic profile and disposal intentions of UK users. Reprod Biomed Online. 2015;31:239–45.
17. Hodes-Wertz B, Druckenmiller S, Smith M, Noyes N. Tick tock: can the clock be stopped? The use of elective oocyte cryopreservation (EOC) as a means to preserve fertility (PF). Fertil Steril. 2013;98:S235.
18. Nekkebroeck J, Stoop D, Devroey P. O-036 A preliminary profile of women opting for oocyte cryopreservation for non-medical reasons. Hum Reprod. 2010;25:i14–7.
19. Lampic C, Svanberg AS, Karlstrom P, Tyden T. Fertility awareness, intentions concerning childbearing, and attitudes towards parenthood among female and male academics. Hum Reprod. 2006;21:558–64.
20. Maheshwari A, Porter M, Shetty A, Bhattacharya S. Women's awareness and perceptions of delay in childbearing. Fertil Steril. 2008;90:1036–42.
21. Bonneux L, Zaadstra BM, De Beer JAA. Sensible family planning: de not get children too late but not too early either. Ned Tijdschr Geneeskd. 2008;152:1507–12.
22. Good I, Savulescu J. In favour of freezing eggs for non-medical reasons. Bioethics. 2009;23:47–58.
23. Dondorp WJ, de Wert G. Fertility preservation for healthy women: ethical aspects. Hum Reprod. 2009;24:1779–85.
24. Mertes H. The portrayal of healthy women requesting oocyte cryopreservation. Facts Views Vis Obgyn. 2013;5:141–6.
25. Mertes H. Does company-sponsored egg freezing promote or confine women's reproductive autonomy? J Assist Reprod Genet. 2015;32:1205–9.
26. Stoop D, Maes E, Polyzos NP, Verheyen G, Tournaye H, Nekkebroeck J. Does oocyte banking for anticipated gamete exhaustion influence future relational and reproductive choices? A follow-up of bankers and non-bankers. Hum Reprod. 2015;30:338–44.
27. Knopman JM, Noyes N, Grifo JA. Cryopreserved oocytes can serve as the treatment for secondary infertility: a novel model for egg donation. Fertil Steril. 2010;93:2413.e7–e9.
28. Wyverkens E, et al. The meaning of the sperm donor for heterosexual couples: confirming the position of the father. Fam Process. 2015;56(1):203–16.
29. Mertes H, Pennings G. Social egg freezing: for better, not for worse. Reprod Biomed Online. 2011;23:824–9.
30. Garcia-Velasco JA, Domingo J, Cobo A, Martínez M, Carmona L, Pellicer A. Five years' experience using oocyte vitrification to preserve fertility for medical and nonmedical indications. Fertil Steril. 2013;99:1994–9.

31. Cil AP, Bang H, Oktay K. Age-specific probability of live-birth with oocyte cryopreservation: an individual patient data meta-analysis. Fertil Steril. 2013;100:492–9.
32. Gold E, Copperman K, Witkin G, Jones C, Copperman AB. Fertil Steril. 2006;3:S201.
33. Klein J, Howard M, Grunfeld L, Mukherjee T, Sandler B, Copperman AB. P-486: preliminary experience of an oocyte cryopreservation program: are patients presenting too late? Fertil Steril. 2006;86:S315.
34. Sage CFF, Kolb BM, Treiser SL, Silverberg KM, Barritt J, Copperman A. Oocyte cryopreservation in women seeking elective fertility preservation—a multicenter analysis. Obstet Gynecol. 2008;111:20S.
35. Vallejo V, Lee JA, Schuman L, Witkin G, Cervantes E, Sandler B, Copperman A. Social and psychological assessment of women undergoing elective oocyte cryopreservation: a 7-year analysis. Open J Obstetric Gynecol. 2013;3(1):1–7. doi: 10.4236/ojog.2013.31001.
36. Mertes H, Pennings G. Elective oocyte cryopreservation: who should pay? Hum Reprod. 2012;27:9–13.

Index

© Springer International Publishing Switzerland 2018
D. Stoop (ed.), *Preventing Age Related Fertility Loss*,
DOI 10.1007/978-3-319-14857-1

O

MIX
Papier aus verantwortungsvollen Quellen
Paper from responsible sources
FSC® C105338

If you have any concerns about our products,
you can contact us on
ProductSafety@springernature.com

In case Publisher is established outside the EU,
the EU authorized representative is:
Springer Nature Customer Service Center GmbH
Europaplatz 3, 69115 Heidelberg, Germany

Printed by Libri Plureos GmbH
in Hamburg, Germany